HOW TO PROLONG LIFE :

AN ENQUIRY INTO

THE CAUSE OF "OLD AGE"

AND

"NATURAL DEATH"

Showing the Diet and Agents best adapted for a Lengthened Prolongation of Human Life on Earth.

Rejuvenescence : By means of Phosphorus & Distilled Water.

BY

C. DE LACY EVANS, M.R.C.S.E., Ph.D.

Solly Medalist, St. Thomas's Hospital,
Late Surgeon St. Saviour's Hospital, Surgeon Gold Coast of Africa, an
Hon. Surgeon to Lady Sandhurst's Home.

CHAS. J. SAWYER, LTD.,
23, NEW OXFORD ST.,
LONDON, W.C.
1910.

THIS WORK IS

Dedicated

TO

SIR ISAAC HOLDEN, BART.,

AS A TOKEN OF ADMIRATION

FOR THE INTEREST HE FOR YEARS HAS TAKEN

IN THE SUBJECTS OF

DIET AND LONGEVITY,

AND IN RECOGNITION OF HIS MANY EFFORTS

TO POPULARISE,

BY PRECEPT AND EXAMPLE,

MANY OF THE IDEAS CONTAINED HEREIN.

Reprinted 1971
By

Health Research
PO Box 850
Pomeroy, WA 99347
www.healthresearchbooks.com
publish@pomeroy-wa.com
Phone: 509-843-2385

CONTENTS.

	PAGE
PREFACE	xi

CHAPTER I.
THE CAUSE OF "OLD AGE" AND "NATURAL DEATH" . 19

CHAPTER II.
THE SOURCE OF THE ACCUMULATIONS WHICH CAUSE "OLD AGE" AND "NATURAL DEATH" . . 51

CHAPTER III.
DIET IN COMPOSITION AND QUANTITY AS BEST ADAPTED TO A PROLONGED EXISTENCE 69

CHAPTER IV.
INSTANCES OF LONGEVITY IN MAN AND IN THE ANIMAL AND VEGETABLE KINGDOMS 123

CHAPTER V.
THE PREVENTION OF DISEASE 165

CHAPTER VI.
AGENTS BEST ADAPTED FOR A LENGTHENED PROLONGATION OF EXISTENCE 177

CHAPTER VII.
CONCLUSION	 209
APPENDIX	 221
GLOSSARY	 225

PREFACE

"If my abilities were equal to my wishes, there should be neither pain nor poverty in the universe."—ADDISON.

IN every being throughout animated Nature, from the most insignificant insect to the most enlightened, ennobled, and highly developed human being, we notice a deeply rooted love for one possession before all others, and that is the possession of *Life*. What will not a man give to preserve his life? What would he not give to prolong it? The value of riches, titles, honour, power, and worldly prospects are as nought compared with the value which every sane man, however humble, and even miserable, places on the preservation of his life.

Human life, physically considered, is a chemical animal operation; and, whatever it may be as an abstract principle, the manifestations and phenomena of life are dependent upon matter in a state of change by the united powers of Nature, and are embodied in a few elementary and grand physical and chemical processes.

The laws of life and of death, looked upon in this light, form the basis of a fixed science—the MACROBIOTIC, or the art of prolonging life.

There is, however, a distinction to be made between this art and the science of medicine, but the one is auxiliary to the other.

There is a state of body which we term *health*; *plus* or *minus* divergences from this path we call *disease*. The object of medicine is to guide these variations to a given centre of bodily equilibrium; but the object of the macrobiotic art is by the founding of dietetic and other rules, on general principles, to preserve the body in health, and thereby prolong life.

In the present work the author has attempted to go beyond this, by inquiring into the *causes* which have a share in producing the changes which are observed as age advances, and, further, by pointing out a means of checking them.

"He who writes, or speaks, or meditates, without

facts as landmarks to his understanding, is like a mariner cast on the wide ocean, without a compass or a rudder to his ship." If he conceives an idea, a phantom of his own imagination, and attempts to make it a reality, by accepting only those facts or phenomena which accord with his premature conception, ignoring those which contradict this shadow or idea, but which may nevertheless be demonstrably true, he creates a *theory* which may be incorrect, and if so it is doomed, sooner or later, to destruction. Although it possibly required but a few hours to construct, centuries may elapse before it is finally destroyed. The founder of an erroneous hypothesis creates a *monster*, which only serves to combat and stifle *Truth*. The struggle can last for a time only, for Truth must of necessity ultimately prevail.

" The true philosopher always seeks to explain and illustrate Nature by means of *facts*, of phenomena, that is, by experiments, the devising and discovery of which is his task, and by which he causes the object of his investigation to speak as it were intelligibly to him; but it is by carefully observing and arranging all such facts as are in connection with it, that insight into its nature is attained. For we must never forget that *every phenomenon has its reason, every effect its cause.*"—BACON.

"The history of science gives us the consoling assurance that we shall succeed, by pursuing the path of experiment and observation, in unveiling the mysteries of organic life, and that we shall be enabled to obtain decided, definite answers to the question—What are *causes* which have a share in producing vital phenomena?"—LIEBIG.

"Let no man be alarmed at the multitude of the objects presented to his attention; for it is this, on the contrary, which ought rather to awaken hope. . . If there were anyone amongst us who, when interrogated respecting the objects of Nature, was always prepared to answer by *facts*, the discovery of causes and the foundation of all sciences would be the work of a few years."—BACON.

The purpose of the author is to make known the results of inquiries into the causes of what is termed the "decay of nature," not theoretically or by accepting only those facts which accord with a preconceived idea, but by collecting all facts bearing on the subject, and making clear and straightforward deductions therefrom.

It is not written for the purpose of conveying a signification of man's individual greatness, nor of ignoring a Supreme Being. It is our increasing knowledge of the phenomena of Nature, and the laws by which they are regulated, which makes us conscious of, and teaches us to recognise, the perfection, the greatness, and unfathomable wisdom of an all-wise CREATOR, whose works and actions become daily more manifest in their illimitable impressions, the sublimity and greatness of which the human mind is not capable of conceiving. The most untiring imagination—the most exalted mind —will contemplate images and fashion forms, which, when compared with reality, appear but as bubbles of brilliant and changing colours—to vanish, leaving the contemplator in forced recognition of his own frailties and imperfections, but not enlightened on the inscrutable wisdom of an infinitely higher Being.

This work is founded upon a paper on "Ossification the Cause of 'Old Age,'" read by the author before the St. Thomas's Hospital Medical and Physical Society, on October 26, 1876.

The author first conceived the idea of the possible prolongation of existence, from a publication entitled

Patriarchal Longevity, by "Parallax," in which ossification as a cause of old age was first pointed out, and from which several quotations are given; many of the instances of longevity are taken from *Records of Longevity*, by Easton and Bailey, and Hufeland's *Art of Prolonging Life*, edited by the late Sir Erasmus Wilson, F.R.S.

Regarding the analyses of foods, at Sir Isaac Holden's suggestion, I intend shortly to publish them, in a separate form, as nothing has as yet been written which gives the relative *solubility* and *insolubility* of the *ashes* which they contain, which is so important to this subject. A glossary of scientific terms is appended.

It has long been the opinion of scientific men, that by suitable diet and regularity, the blessings of life may be enjoyed in fair health to a "green old age." The purpose of this work is to show that we may for a time curb the *causes* which are visible in *effect* as age advances, and thus prolong life, and further, that by other means, founded upon simple fact, we may accomplish this for a lengthened period.

Sir Benjamin Ward Richardson recently said: "Presuming human beings are born of good and wholesome constitution, they are, except for accidental destructive agencies, in a fair way to live five times their maturity, that is, five times 21 years, the natural term of the anatomical life, namely, 105 years, a term few reach, but which is attainable as a matter of experience, and so attainable, as a matter of natural law, that the majority of men and women would attain it if they lived properly."

Dr. Kearney, in an article on the subject of this work in the *Transatlantic Monthly*, stated that there was no reason why human life should not be extended to at least 200 years; and many other writers are of similar opinions.

The chemistry of the present—not to predict the future—points distinctly, ultimately, to more than this.

Artemus Ward gave sound advice when he wrote, " Never prophesy *unless* you know."

Chemistry does not require a prophet. It is an experimental and true science, founded on fact, not upon fiction.

When we consider that the difference between an old man and a young one is due to the gradual accumulation of certain definite and simple chemical compounds, which cause an alteration in appearance, structure, and function, there is no reason why eventually—perhaps shortly—we should not have these changes under our *control*, to such an extent that accident alone would be the enemy. Furthermore, the chemist of the future may—aye, will—succeed in preparing an artificial diet, which will contain the elements alone required for nutrition, without those which are pernicious to longevity, and cause both the characteristics of age and untimely death. Science does not contradict the approach of a period when—for some at all events—lost Arcadia may be regained, and when, as Sir Walter Scott wrote, " Sages shall become monarchs of the earth; and death itself retreat from their frown."

C. DE LACY EVANS.

17, NUTFORD PLACE,
MARBLE ARCH,
W.

HOW TO PROLONG LIFE

CHAPTER I.

THE CAUSE OF "OLD AGE" AND "NATURAL DEATH."

WITH all our physiological, anatomical, and philosophical discoveries, there are left many questions at present not solved; amongst others, the action of the brain, thought, motion, life, and the possible prolongation of existence.

"Nature speaks to us in a peculiar language, in the language of phenomena. She answers at all times questions which are put to her; and such questions are experiments."

In "old age" the body differs materially from youth, in actions, sensibility, function, and composition. The active, fluid, sensitive, and elastic body of youth gradually gives place to *induration*, rigidity, and *decrepitude*, which terminate in "natural death."

In Nature there are distinct reasons for every change, for development, growth, decomposition, and death.

If with our minds free from theory, and unbiassed by *hypotheses*, we ask Nature the cause of these changes, she will surely answer us. Let us ask her the cause of these differences between youth and old age—why the various functions of the body gradually cease; why we become "old" and die.

The most marked feature in old age is that a *fibrinous, gelatinous*, and earthy deposit has taken place in the system; the latter being composed chiefly of phosphate and carbonate of lime, with small quantities of sulphate of lime, magnesia, and traces of other earths.

Among physiologists and medical philosophers generally, the idea prevails that the "*ossification*" (or the gradual accumulation of earthy salts in the system) which characterises "natural death," is the *result* of "old age," but investigation shows that such an explanation is unsatisfactory. For in the first place, if "old age" (which is really the number of years a person has lived) is the cause of the ossification which accompanies it, then, if "like causes produce like effects," *all* of the same age should be found in the same state of ossification; but investigation proves beyond all doubt that such is not the case. How common it is to see individuals about fifty years old, as aged and decrepit as others at seventy or eighty!

We will first inquire into the differences found by investigation between youth and old age, in the many structures and organs of the body.

Bone.—The average constituents of bone at about the prime of life, according to an analysis by Berzelius, are:

Organic matter, gelatine and bloodvessels		33·30
	Phosphate of lime	51·04
Inorganic	Carbonate of lime	11·30
or	Fluoride of calcium	2·00
Earthy matter	Phosphate of magnesia	1·16
	Soda and chloride of sodium	1·20
		100·00

Thus we see that 66·7 per cent., or about two-thirds, are composed of *inorganic* or earthy compounds. The organic or gelatinous portion contains about 10 per cent. of water (if recent).

Compact bony substance contains more earthy matter than the spongy bone; and, proportionally, more phosphate of lime to the carbonate than the latter.

If we take the bones of a *child*, of a *young man* in the prime of life, and of an *old man*, and subject a given weight of each of them to a simple analysis, the earthy constituents of which may be easily obtained by subjecting them to a strong heat, with free access of air, by which means the animal or organic matter is entirely consumed, the earthy part remaining, and carefully weigh the residue of earthy salts, chiefly lime, what do we find?

That the bones of the child contain a certain amount of earthy compounds (according to its age); that the bones of the young man contain a larger proportion of earthy compounds than those of the child, and that the bones of the old man contain a larger proportion than either. If we also take the stages intermediate between childhood and manhood, on the one hand, and manhood and old age on the other, we obtain the same result, clearly showing that *from some cause the amount of earthy compounds in the bones gradually increases from birth to old age.*

"Accordingly to Schreger and others, there is a considerable increase in the earthy constituents of bones with advancing years. Dr. Rees states that this is especially marked in the long bones and the bones of the head, which, in the fœtus, do not contain the excess of earthy matter found in those of the adult. . . . Thus in the child, where the animal matter predominates, it is not uncommon to find, after an injury to the bones, that they become bent, or only partially broken, from the large amount of flexible animal matter which they contain. Again also in aged people, where the bones contain a large proportion of earthy matter, the animal matter at the same time being deficient in quantity and quality, the bones are more brittle, their elasticity is destroyed, and hence fracture takes place more readily."—GRAY.

From *embryonic* life to birth a gradual process of ossification is going on, and even at birth the *epiphyses* of most of the cylindrical bones, all the bones of the *carpus*, the five smaller ones of the *tarsus*, the *patella*, *sesamoid* bones, and the last pieces of the *coccyx* are still unossified.

From birth this process of ossification still continuing, the epiphyses become united to their shafts, the ossific centres of the *vertebræ* and cranium gradually join to form their respective bones, and it is not till about the thirtieth year that the full development of the bones of the skeleton is attained. From the prime of life we trace onward this gradual process of ossification; the *inter-vertebral* cartilages become shrunken, hard, and inelastic, causing in old age diminished stature and an inclination to bend forwards; in some instances the sutures of the cranium are gradually obliterated, and the once separate bones unite; the cartilages of the ribs, and articular ends of bones harden and ossify; the bones of the sternum unite; from loss of teeth changes are observed in the shape of the lower jaw; the segments of the *hyoid* bone become united together, forming in old age a single bone; the *cartilages* of the larynx become ossified; even the *ligaments* of joints become so hardened, that their former pliability is usurped by the limited, awkward, and decrepid movements of old age.

Thus we find that the bones at this period of life contain proportionately more earthy matter than those in youth.

Muscles.—As age advances the muscles diminish in bulk, the fibres become rigid and less *contractile*, becoming paler or even yellowish in colour, and are not influenced by *stimuli* to the same extent as in youth.

Tendons and adjacent portions of muscular tissue and *aponeuroses* become hardened and even ossified.

There is also a diminution in the fluid in the sheaths of the tendons.

If we analyse a given weight of muscular tissue taken from an *old* man, and the same weight taken from a *young* man, we find that the former contains more earthy matter than the latter. Any structure or organ of the body will give the same result, *i.e.*, that there exists throughout the system more earthy matter in old age than in *adolescence*, and that this earthy matter has been gradually accumulating from the first stage of existence.

Brain.—We will next briefly consider the alterations in the brain and nerve centres in old age.

The brain—the organ which presides over every thought and action of our material bodies, which constitutes one of the great central masses of the nervous system, and which is in constant telegraphic communication with every structure and part of the body, through the medium of the spinal column and nerves, the latter of which are so wonderfully distributed by their minute *ramifications*, that there is not a point on the whole surface of the body, the size of a pin's head, which we could wound, without the brain being at once cognisant of the fact—differs from most other organs and structures of the body in containing phosphorus, in an *unoxidised* form, upon which subject we will treat hereafter.

The brain grows or increases in size up to about forty years of age, when it reaches its maximum weight. After this period there is a gradual and slow diminution in weight of about one ounce in every ten years.

According to Cazanvieilh, the longitudinal diameter of the brain of an *old man*, compared with that of a *young man*, is six inches one line, French measure, for the former, and six inches four lines for the latter; whilst the transverse diameter is four inches ten lines in the *old man*, and five inches in the *young man*. The same authority gives the following comparative measurements of different parts of the brain at the three periods of life, puberty, prime of life, and old age:

	PERSONS AT PUBERTY.		PRIME OF LIFE.		OLD AGE.	
	in.	lns.	in.	lns.	in.	lns.
Thal. optica	1	5½	1	6	1	4½
Corp. striata	2	6	2	6	2	4½
Corp. callosum	3	4½	3	5	2	7
Mesocephalon { length	0	10	0	11	0	10½
{ breadth	1	0	1	1	1	0
Cerebellum { length	2	2	2	3	2	3
{ breadth	3	9	3	9	3	9

Thus it appears that with the exception of the cerebellum (or animal brain), every part of the encephalon diminishes in size in old age. Further, the convolutions of the brain become less and less distinct and prominent.

Membranes of the Brain.—The *dura mater* is often found apparently collapsed or corrugated, particularly in the very aged, when little fluid is found beneath it; it is frequently found to be thickened and indurated, and ossific deposits on the arachnoid surface are very common. These are generally described as resulting from a chronic inflammatory action, but where during life there have been no symptoms of any inflammatory disease, we must put it down as concomitant to "old age," or that gradual process of ossification which either accompanies or causes such a state of the system.

Thickening and opacity of the *arachnoid* are often found in old people, the fluid secreted being sometimes turbid and albuminous; the membrane is sometimes found to have an *abnormal* dryness, and osseous deposits sometimes, though rarely, occur; but a roughness or grittiness, giving the sensation of fine sand under the finger, is more often met with, this roughness being due to earthy deposits. The choroid plexus is sometimes in a varicose state, and the membranes lining the ventricles are found thick and opaque.

We now come to the most important change of all, which fully accounts for the many differences in the brain existing between youth and old age, that is, the changes in the bloodvessels supplying it. The arteries in old age become thickened and lessened in calibre from fibrinous, gelatinous, and earthy deposits. This is more easily detected in the larger vessels; but all, even to the most minute subdivisions, undergo the same gradual change. Thus the supply of blood to the brain becomes less and less; hence the diminu-

THE CAUSE OF "OLD AGE." 27

tion in size of the organ from the prime of life to old age; hence the functions of the brain become gradually impaired; the vigorous brain of middle life gradually giving place to loss of memory, confusion of ideas, inability to follow a long current of thought, notions oblivious of the past and regardless as to the future, carelessness of momentary impressions, softening of the brain, and that imbecility so characteristic of extreme age.

In the brain, "the arteries most commonly found ossified are the internal carotids and the basilar; but the circle of Willis, and the vessels departing from it, as well as the arterial ramifications which appear between the convolutions, and come out upon the surface, often participate more or less in this morbid state. Cartilaginous degeneration is still more extensive, and seems to precede the ossific deposits. Cartilaginous and ossific formations in the coats of arteries of the brain occasion irregular distribution of blood, and interrupted or imperfect supplies of this fluid to some parts of the organ, disposing to aneurismal dilatations, to rupture, and consequently to the production of apoplexy and paralysis."—COPLAND.

"*Ossification* is detected (with the naked eye) only in the *arteries;* but it occurs in them very frequently and to a very great extent, particularly in advanced life."—*Ibid.*

"*After the age of fifty*, the walls of the bloodvessels are very liable to 'degeneration.' The aorta, in particular, becomes dilated, the elasticity of its walls impaired, and its inner surface roughened by large, irregular, whitish, elevated patches of morbid matter, lying immediately beneath a superficial layer of the inner coat, and composed of a mixture of *earthy and fatty matter*. . . . In the *smaller* arteries, the ossification proceeds much more uniformly, and they become at last more or less completely converted into *smooth bony tubes*. The capillaries are equally liable with the arteries to degeneration."—HOOPER'S *Physician's Vade Mecum.*

"The cerebral arteries of old persons are frequently found studded with cartilaginous and osseous laminæ."

"The ossification of arteries has been ascribed by many authors to *slight* chronic inflammatory action. The experiments of M. Rayer and M. Cruveilheir seem to confirm this inference, as an *occasional* occurrence at least, particularly in the fibrous and cartilaginous structures, artificially excited, being generally followed by ossiform depositions; but in a number of cases, particularly in those where the deposit takes place in the cellular tissues, *no inflammatory action can be detected* previously to this change; besides, increased vascular action frequently exists, without being attended with ossiform depositions. This lesion, therefore, cannot be altogether ascribed to this cause, although frequently resulting from it in a certain order of tissues. It would be correct to consider it merely as a consequence of disorder of the *natural* process of nutrition and secretion. . . . But *to what cause* is this disorder of the nutritive function to be imputed, particularly when it occurs in parts which have *not evinced any sign of inflammatory action*, as in the cellular tissue connecting the internal coats of *arteries?* The importance of this inquiry may appear, from the *very great proportion of persons in advanced years* who are affected in some organ or tissue with this lesion, and from the remarkable part it performs in the production of a number of diseases of the most dangerous description."—COPLAND'S *Med. Dic.* art. " Arteries."

MM. Rostan, Recamier, and others, agree in considering that softening of the brain is occasionally unconnected with any inflammatory action, *particularly in aged persons.*

We have quoted from the above authorities to show that ossification and thickening of the arteries of the brain has not been overlooked, but that it is a fact which has been known for many years; also to show that this gradual process of ossification is not due to any inflammatory action. And we shall show that this earthy matter has been deposited from the blood, and increases year by year with old age, thus lessening the calibre of the larger vessels, partially, and in some cases, fully, "clogging up" the capillaries, gradually diminishing the supply of blood to the brain, causing its diminution in size in old age, and fully accounting for the gradual loss of the mental capabilities before enumerated.

As age advances, the energies of the *ganglial system*

decline; digestion, circulation, and the secretory functions are lessened; the *ganglia* diminish in size, become firmer, and of a deeper hue. In old age the *nerves* become tougher and firmer, the medullary substance diminishes, and their bloodvessels lessen in calibre. The sensibility of the whole cerebro-spinal system decreases, hence diminution of the intellectual powers, lessened activity and strength in the organs of locomotion in advanced age.

Another important and striking fact is that the brain of an old man contains a less amount of phosphorus than that of a younger man.

Arteries.—As with the arteries of the brain, the same process of gradual ossification extends to every vessel, the arborescent ramifications of which supply, without exception, every part of the system.* Bichat and Baillee considered that the larger proportion of persons above sixty years of age have some part of the arterial system affected by these depositions.

Veins.—In old age the *vasa vasorum* decrease and become indistinct, the arteries lessen in calibre, they therefore hold a less amount of blood than in younger life; the pressure is thrown on the veins, which dilate, their coats becoming thinner, and they become tortuous or even varicose.

Hearts.—In the heart "the coronary arteries are

* Dr. C. J. B. Williams, F.R.S., speaking of calcareous degenerations, observes: "This process is therefore to be viewed as almost entirely of a chemical nature, and as consisting in the concretion and accumulation of calcareous salts, phosphate and carbonate of lime in the debris of animal matter."

frequently ossified, both in their trunks and in their subdivisions." In many cases this ossification is not visible; but, on analysing the same weight of muscular tissue taken from the heart of two individuals at different stages of life, we find the same excess of earthy matter in old age as we did in other structures already considered; the capillaries gradually diminish in calibre, the muscular fibres of the organ are improperly nourished, the fibres become paler in colour, the cavities dilated and their walls thinned, in some cases becoming more or less hardened or indurated, in others giving away to fatty degeneration. The valves also undergo cartilaginous and osseous transformations. The supply of blood to the organ is gradually diminished, and its feeble contractions impel the blood along vessels already indurated and ossified, to organs which have undergone the same degree of ossification, and are therefore unable to properly perform their necessary functions.

"About the age of forty, and still more so as the age of fifty is approached, the sanguineous circulation becomes more and more languid, particularly in the veins; hence the frequency of venous congestions and visceral obstructions, with various diseases depending thereon, particularly hæmorrhoids, bilious derangements, bilious and gastric fevers, inflammations, affections of the heart, apoplexy and paralysis, derangements of the stomach and liver, hæmatemesis, affections of the joints, as gout and rheumatism; diseases of the urinary organs, hysteria and uterine disorders, hypochondriasis, and affections of the mind."—COOPER.

Lungs.—The *lungs* gradually lose their elasticity and increase in density; the air cells and bronchi become dilated; hence emphysema and chronic bronchitis, so often seen in the very aged.

We now come to the organs of *secretion* and *digestion*.

Salivary Glands.—To commence with the *salivary glands*. We find that they are hardened and ossified; their bulk in many cases decreases with age; the saliva is either secreted in so small a quantity that food is only partially moistened in the mouth, and swallowed with difficulty, or it is secreted in large quantities, running, or 'dribbling,' continually from the mouth in the very aged, its composition being altered in containing more water than normal.

Stomach.—In the stomach, the gastric juice (the use of which is to dissolve the various kinds of foods, reducing the albuminous and fibrinous portions of it to a state fit for absorption into the system) is secreted in a diluted form, and is deficient in pepsin; thus the first process of digestion is improperly carried out. Moreover, the muscular walls of the stomach gradually lose their wonted contractility, the peristaltic motions become weak, and the chyme, or product of the gastric digestion, is feebly transmitted through the pyloric orifice to the intestinal tube, instead of passing in a more vigorous manner, as it does in the prime of life.

Liver.—The *liver*, besides effecting important changes in certain constituents of the blood during its circulation through the gland, is also the secreting organ by which the *bile* is formed. The bile is separated from the blood by the hepatic cell, and is discharged into small ducts, which unite, and terminate in the *ductus communis choledochus*. In old age the minute bloodvessels become hardened and diminished in calibre; the hepatic cells become indurated, and therefore their secretion becomes slightly altered; but this alteration differs in degree according to the amount of venous congestion, so often met with in advanced life, and which is caused by the induration, or hardening, of the organ, not allowing that amount of dilatation which existed in the earlier periods of life.

"Diseases of the liver very seldom occur until after puberty." But in after-life how few are free from some congestive or structural disorder of the organ! In childhood and youth the organ possesses sufficient elasticity to allow any increased flow of blood to pass, but in old age the hardened and ossified tunnels will not and cannot dilate; the veins of the abdomen and lower limbs receive the pressure, and become varicose.

In old age fatty matters are not thoroughly emulsified, or absorbed by the lacteals; this may be due to an alteration in the fluid secreted by the *pancreas*.

Intestines.—In the intestines the small vessels which supply the follicles and various glands become indurated, or even "clogged up," in old age; the walls of the intestines become opaque, and lose their contractility; the *villi* containing the *lacteals* undergo the same gradual alteration, the latter of which having coats which year by year become less pervious, less and less nourishment is absorbed into the system. From these alterations in the digestive organs, we see, firstly, that food is improperly digested; secondly, that the chyle, or nutrient part of it, is only partially absorbed by the lacteals; further, that these defects of function are caused by a gradual process of induration and ossification.

Testes.—In old age the *testes* shrink and nearly disappear; the spermatic fluid is altered in composition and gradually lost, whilst from a gradual induration and ossification, the vessels of the *erectile* tissues no longer admitting of dilatation, the function of the latter as such is lost.

As age advances, the *prostate* gland is disposed to become enlarged; and "its ducts often contain small rounded concretions, about the size of a millet-seed, which are composed of carbonate of lime and animal matter."

Cowper's glands appear to diminish in old age.

Uterus.—"From the gradual *effects* of *age* alone, independent of impregnation, the uterus shrinks, and becomes paler in colour and *harder in texture;* its triangular form is lost; the body and neck become less distinguishable from each other; the orifices become less characteristic."—QUAIN.

Ovaries.—The same consolidation applies to the *ovaries*, in which Dr. Martin Barry has shown a *large number* of microscopic ovisacs to exist. Nevertheless, the Graafian vesicles approach the surface of the ovary and burst, the ovum and fluid contents of the vesicle passing into the Fallopian tube, *periodically*, from about fifteen only, up to about forty-five to fifty years of age, after which period of life, owing to a hardened and ossified state of the ovary, the vesicles are unable to approach the surface of the organ ; *they exist*, but they are imprisoned, their development is arrested, they shrink or disappear ; the powers of regeneration and reproduction are therefore lost.

The *urinary organs* are modified by the same consolidation. In the tubuli uriniferi and pelvis of the kidney, calculi are frequently found. The bladder becomes firmer, thicker, and less elastic in old age.

In old age, *adipose* and *cellular tissues* are changed. Fatty matters diminish in quantity, become more fluid and deeper in colour. Cellular tissue gradually becomes denser, more fragile, and inelastic, sometimes assuming a fibrous character.

Serous membranes become denser, and ossific deposits are often found in them; their surface also becomes drier in old age than in youth.

Fibrous structures become firmer, tougher, and more rigid, and often ossified.

In old age fibrin and gelatin increase ; albumen diminishes. Many secretions become acrid and irritating, and mucous fluid generally increased.

Owing to languor of the circulation and decreased nerve power, the generation of *animal heat* is diminished, although exhalation and evaporation from the lungs and skin, both of which lower the temperature of the body, are not so great in degree in old age as in youth.

If we inquire into the cause of the senile changes in the organs of sensation, we find that sight gradually fails, that hearing, taste, and smell are gradually altered by the same process of induration and ossification.

Eye.—In the *eye*, in old age, there is diminished secretion of the aqueous fluid in the anterior chamber, the cornea becomes less prominent; the pupil becomes more dilated from lessened nervous sensibility; hence distant sight, and the indistinct and confused view of near objects in the aged.

"Extreme age is a strong predisposing cause to amaurosis."—MIDDLEMORE.

"It is most frequent at and after the middle period of life."—LAWRENCE.

"The state of the retina, when examined after death, in amaurotic eyes, accords with these views . . . it has been found thickened, opaque, spotted, buff-coloured, tough, and in some cases even ossified."—COOPER.

"One case (of amaurosis) very analogous to amblyopia * senilis, is believed to depend upon a

* Amblyopia (from ἀμβλὺς, dull ; ὼψ, the eye). Hippocrates means by this word the dimness of sight to which *old people* are subject.— *Aph.* 31, sect. 3.

diminution of the pigmentum nigrum, which secretion, in some individuals earlier and more considerably, in others later and in a slighter degree, *recedes with other secretions of a different nature.*"—BEER'S *Lehre von den Augenkr.* bk. ii. p. 451.

"In form, colour, degree of transparency, and density, the lens presents marked differences at different periods of life. In the *adult*, the anterior surface of the lens becomes less convex than the posterior, and the substance of the lens firmer (than in childhood), colourless, and transparent. In *old age*, it is flattened on both surfaces, it assumes a yellowish or amber tinge, and is apt to lose its transparency as it gradually increases in toughness and specific gravity."—QUAIN.

"*Old age* may be regarded as one of the predisposing causes to cataract, inasmuch as the disease is most frequent in advanced life."—COOPER.

"If common senile cataract be not caused by death of the lens, if this explanation of its opacity be rejected, we are totally at a loss to explain its frequent occurrence in aged persons. It is evidently *not produced in them by inflammation*, for it takes place first, it is perceived, in the *centre* of the lens; it occurs in old feeble persons, and is *unattended by pain*, or by any morbid effect in the other parts of the eye, which can with propriety be referred to inflammation."—MIDDLEMORE, *Dis. of Eye.*

"On this point, I should say that there is evidence rather of disorganisation, or of alteration in texture, or of a *new deposit* in the lens, than of actual death of it."—COOPER'S *Surg. Dict.* art. "Eye."

"Cataract is often suspected to arise from defective *nutrition* of the lens; some imperfection of the nerve, it is conceived, *may be* concerned."—MACKENZIE.

"The cataract of *old people* generally attacks *both eyes*, within the period of a few months; but in *middle life* we often meet with it in *one eye*, the other having continued unaffected for many years."—MACKENZIE.

In *middle life* cataract may be due to some inflammatory action, and only affect *one eye*, but *true senile cataract* is not caused by death of the lens, is not due to any inflammatory action; but there *is a new deposit* in the lens, which accompanies, or is part of, that gradual induration and ossification found in *old age;* therefore *both* eyes are affected at about the same period.

In old age the cornea becomes altered in shape, hardened, or even opaque; the sclerotic undergoes the same modifications, and in some cases is even found ossified. To show that ossification sometimes exists, and is possible, we quote a few extreme cases.

"Scarpa dissected an eye, which was almost entirely transformed into a *stony substance.* It was taken from the body of an *old woman*, and was not above half as large as the sound one. The cornea appeared dusky, and, behind it, the iris of a singular shape, concave, and without any pupil in its centre. The rest of the eyeball, from the limits of the cornea backwards, was unusually hard to the touch. The particulars of the dissection in this case will be read with interest in Scarpa's treatise on *Diseases of the Eye*. Haller met with a similar case (see *Obs. Pathol. Oper. Min.* obs. 15). Fabricius Hildanus, Lancisi, Morgagni, Morand, Zinn, and Pellier, make distinct mention of calculi in the interior of the eye. Ossification of the capsule of the lens, of that of the vitreous humour, and of, what was supposed to be, the hyaloid membrane, are noticed by Mr. Wardropp."—COOPER, *Surg. Dict.*

Mr. Wardropp also mentions an instance of ossification of the cornea. In this case the whole eye was altered in form, and the cornea was opaque; in it a piece of bone weighing two grains, oval-shaped, hard, and with a smooth surface, was found between its lamellæ; ossification of the choroid coat and retina was also found. According to the same authority, Walter had in his museum a piece of cornea taken from a man sixty years of age, containing a bony mass which was three lines long, two broad, and weighed two grains.

Many of the above cases are undoubtedly the result either of accident or some inflammatory action; we must not, therefore, consider them as a natural formation: but in old age, we have sufficient evidence to show that the whole structure of the eye is slightly altered, that the solid parts are hardened, and even ossified; parts which in the earlier periods of life were transparent, become opaque; owing to senile changes in the bloodvessels, the humours (which are secreted) are slightly altered in quantity, colour, and transparency; further, that the retina loses its sensibility owing to the changes in the brain and nerves, which have been already considered.

These changes in the eye, caused, firstly, by a gradual process of solidification and ossification, secondly, by diminished nervous sensibility, fully account for cataract, amaurosis, and other diseases of the eye, becoming more prevalent after the middle period of life, and still more frequent in old age. On the other hand, on the same principle that some persons are gifted with genius in one form or other, a being may be blessed with organs of sight possessing tone and nervous sensibility higher and greater in degree than those of the majority of mankind, and may live to a good old age "with eye not dim." But even then his sight is not so clear, precise, or perfect, as it was in the earlier periods of life. It has undergone the same alterations as those found in other individuals; these may be slight—it is but a difference in degree.

Ear.—The *ear* is subject to the same gradual process of ossification. The cartilages of the *external ear* become hardened, or even ossified; the ceruminous glands, which secrete the ear-wax, undergo the same alterations which have been observed in other glands; the secretion becomes less, and is altered in quality. The membrana tympani becomes thickened and indurated; the ligaments connecting the ossicles (malleus, incus, and stapes) become hardened— their pliability is lessened; thus vibrations which are already imperfect, owing to induration of the membrana tympani are improperly conveyed by the ossicles across the cavity of the tympanum, by means of the internal ear (the structures and fluids of which have undergone the same process of consolidation[*]), to the auditory nerve, the sensibility of which decreases with the senile changes of the brain. Hence the impaired and confused hearing so often observed in aged persons.

Tongue—Taste.—The tongue, besides being the organ of the special sense of taste, also possesses in a very high degree that of touch; these sensitive powers are confined to the membrane which covers it, the upper surface of which is studded all over with numerous sensitive papillæ; in old age, from a gradual loss of nervous susceptibility, also from induration of the bloodvessels supplying these papillæ, their sensibility is diminished. The whole membrane covering the tongue is hardened and thickened, its surface becomes dry and furrowed, and the sense of taste is diminished.

Smell.—In the nose, like the ear, the cartilages which determine its shape become hardened and even slightly ossified; the power of contraction and expansion of the nostrils during respiration, so often observed in the child, is not utilised. Internally, the Schneiderian or pituitary membrane becomes hard-

[*] Fluid in the internal cavities is diminished, or even absorbed, in old age.

ened and thickened, the vessels supplying it become indurated and lessened in calibre, and the secretion from the glandular follicles either become less, accounting for that dryness of the nose so often observed in the aged, or it becomes watery and increased in quantity, giving rise to symptoms also characteristic of the same. Moreover, the fibres of the *olfactory*, the special nerve of the sense of smell, gradually lose their wonted susceptibility—hence the sense of smell decreases with age; its peculiar power of protecting the luugs from the inhalation of obnoxious gases, and in helping the organs of taste to discriminate the characters of food, is indifferently carried out.

Touch.—We now come to the sense of touch, and as its principal seat is the skin, we will at the same time consider the senile changes in the latter, which is also important as an organ of excretion and absorption.

"The skin consists of two* layers, the derma or cutis vera, and the epidermis or cuticle. On the surface of the former are the sensitive papillæ; and within, or embedded beneath it, are the sweat-glands, hair follicles, and sebaceous glands." The cutis or true skin, consists of two layers, the *corium* and *papillary layer*. The latter contains the expansions of the sensitive nerves, and consists of numerous small, highly sensitive, and vascular eminences, which rise perpendicularly from its surface, forming the essential element of the organ of touch.

* Some authors give three layers—cuticle, rete mucosum, and cutis vera.

The average length of these papillæ is about the one-hundredth of an inch; but they are of larger size, and more fully developed upon the palmar surface of the hands, and the plantar surface of the feet. Each papilla contains one or more nerve-fibres, and in parts where the sense of touch is most highly developed, these nerve-fibres seem to be connected with small oval bodies, termed "tactile corpuscles," which Wagner describes as resembling minute fir-cones, and considers them an apparatus subservient to the sense of touch; and it is yet an open question whether or not these bodies develop electricity, and, acting as independent and separate ganglia, convey impressions to the brain; but it is out of place to enter upon the subject here: we must therefore content ourselves by inquiring into the senile changes in the skin and organs of touch.

In the first place, in old age the sensibility of the nerves is diminished; the capillaries supplying each papilla are gradually lessened in calibre, or even obliterated. From these two causes the sense of touch is not so perfect in old age as in earlier life. Further, as in other glands, the secretion of the sweat and sebaceous glands is diminished; the skin becomes dry, shrunken, and leather-like; it has a cracked or furrowed appearance, especially noticeable where any flexion of joints takes place, or where wasting of the soft part under the skin causes it to "pucker up." Hence the wrinkles of old persons. In old age, the skin contains more earthy salts than in youth.

Teeth.—A human being is provided with two sets of teeth. The first, or temporary set, make their appearance in childhood, and are developed during fœtal life from the mucous membrane covering the edges of the maxillary arches, by means of papillæ, one for each tooth, which become enclosed by means of a convergence and union of the sides of the primitive dental groove. These papillæ, or pulps, are supplied with bloodvessels and nerves. They gradually enlarge and assume the form of the future teeth, when a gradual process of ossification, or the formation of dentine, commences. A thin osseous shell, or cap of dentine, appears on the points of the pulps; this increases, and eventually takes up its whole substance. At the same time the outer surface of the crown becomes covered with enamel, which is formed from a substance lying on the pulp and adapted to its surface; not by secretion, but by a process analogous to ossification, or a deposition of earthy matter; and we have reason to believe that the beautiful arrangement of this earthy matter, as seen in the minute, wavy, branching tubes lying parallel to each other, in the dentine, measuring about one four thousand five hundredth part of an inch in diameter, and the minute hexagonal rods in the enamel, measuring about one five thousand five hundredth part of an inch in diameter, is due to these earthy salts being deposited from minute pre-existing tubules. The same process still continuing, the root, or fang, is formed, elongates, and the tooth cuts the gum about six or seven months after birth, the temporary teeth being completed by the beginning of the third year. The temporary teeth begin to fall out at seven or eight years of age; these are replaced by the permanent teeth, which are likewise developed before birth (with the exception of the last molars), but which during childhood are lodged in pedunculated cells in the bone.

The eruption of the permanent teeth commences at about seven or eight years, and, with the exception of the wisdom teeth, is completed at thirteen or fourteen years, the latter appearing between seventeen and twenty-five. During this time the jaw increases in depth and length.

In the interior of the bony part of each tooth is a cavity, which descends or ascends, as the case may be, into the root, and thereby communicates with the outer surface. It contains a delicate vascular membrane, which is called the pulp of the tooth, and is supplied with bloodvessels and nerves; and although the bloodvessels send no branches into the hard substance of the teeth, the tubules of the dentine imbibe and convey nutrient fluid to it. In support of this the teeth are often stained yellow in jaundice; and in *young* animals fed on madder, the dentine is often tinged with its colour, but in *older* animals under the same circumstances this colouring does not take place.

As age advances, the bloodvessels supplying the pulp of the teeth indurate and lessen in calibre; earthy matter increases in the cavity of the tooth, which cavity therefore decreases in size, in old teeth becoming almost obliterated. The blood supply to the tooth is gradually cut off, little by little it loses its nourishment; its crown becomes worn away by the almost constant process of mastication; it is not replaced by growth from the root; the tooth decays, and falls out.

Hair.—Hair is made up of an outer, cortical, horny, or fibrous substance, which invests it, and an inner medullary, or pith-like substance, within; the latter is made up of a series of cells, filled with pigment; the bulb, or root, is inserted into the skin in what is termed a hair *follicle*, at the bottom of which is a small vascular eminence—a papilla, by means of which material is supplied for the production and constant growth of the hair, blastema being thrown out, in which nucleated cells arise; these flatten out, unite, and form the fibres which compose the fibrous part of the hair. Many of these cells contain pigment, which gives the different characteristic shades to the hair. Thus one hair grows, is nourished and coloured from the blood, through the agency and powers of selection of a single papilla.

Whatever tends to lessen or cut off the supply of blood to this papilla, robs the hair of its powers of growth, nourishment, and colour. During thought, hard study, or mental worry, there is an increased flow of blood to the brain at the expense of that supplying the surface; the hair loses, at all events temporarily, part of its nourishment; hence prema-

THE CAUSE OF "OLD AGE."

ture greyness and baldness. Again, during fright, owing to intense contractions of the bloodvessels caused by the action of the sympathetic nerves, the supply of blood is taken away from these papillæ supplying the hair; by this means many persons have become grey, or even partially bald, in a single night. But there is another important change which we have to consider—that is, the process of induration and ossification, which gradually lessens, or even entirely obstructs, the supply of blood to these papillæ, by which means the hair, little by little, loses its powers of growth, nourishment, and colour.

Thus in old age the hair is no longer nourished, it loses its colour—becomes grey or white, for lack of pigment; some of the papillæ are even totally deprived of their blood supply; therefore the bulb shrivels and shrinks, the hair falls away.

In the foregoing pages we have pointed out the differences existing between youth and old age. In the former the various organs and structures are elastic, yielding, and pliable; the senses are keen, the mind active. In the latter, these qualities are usurped by hardness, rigidity, and ossification; the senses are wanting in susceptibility, the mind in memory and capacity.

Further, that these changes are due, firstly, to a gradual accumulation of fibrinous and gelatinous substances; secondly, to a gradual deposition of earthy compounds, chiefly phosphate and carbonate of lime. These, acting in concert, diminish the calibre of the larger arterial vessels, and by degrees partially, and sometimes fully, obliterate the capillaries. By these depositions every organ and structure in the system is altered in density and function; the fluid, elastic, pliable, and active state of body gives place to a solid, inactive, rigid, ossified, and decrepit condition. The whole system is "choked up"; the curtain falls, the play of life is ended, terminating in so-called "natural death."

The general impression is that this accumulation of fibrinous, gelatinous, and osseous matter, is the *result* of old age—the result of time, the remote *effects* of the failure of that mysterious animal principle—life. But in an after chapter we shall show that this great vital principle, which is centred in the cerebro-spinal axis, gradually wanes, because the brain and nerves by degrees lose their supply of blood, their powers of selection and imbibition, and are deprived of their ordained nourishment by means of this gradual process of induration and ossification.

Another prevailing idea is that the embryo, at its first period of existence, is endowed with a certain allotment of vitality—of life, the powers of which perfect the organs and structures of the body, and gradually decline, exhausting itself till death, and that the greater the amount and degree of the numerous uses it is put to, the sooner and more rapidly will existence collapse. The more luminous the flame, the sooner will it be extinguished!

THE CAUSE OF "OLD AGE."

To this idea there are many objections, which would cause us to throw it aside. In many diseases how often is the sunbeam of life, nearly extinguished, known to recover, and shine again, perhaps more brilliantly than before! If we ask its source, can parents, whose supply of vitality is decreasing, give more than they possess to their offspring, and yet keep a portion to themselves?

Vitality emanates from the parent, but there is no doubt that instead of experiencing a diminution, it increases up to a certain period of life, when its maximum grade is attained, after which period the manifestations and functions of life gradually decline. For this decline Nature gives a reason, and tells man it is in his power to arrest and curb the causes.

Every organ and structure of the body, up to a certain period of life, possesses, *per se*, the power of reproducing any waste in structure or composition, under favourable circumstances; but after this period, the bloodvessels, which supply without exception every part of the body, become so indurated, hardened, and ossified, that their powers of irrigating and nourishing the different structures decline; the waste is therefore greater than the renewal.

By a simple method of inquiry, we have asked the cause of the differences between youth and old age —why the various functions of the body are taken away; why we become old and die.

Nature has answered us.

Induration and ossification are the *causes* of "*old age*" and "*natural death*." And upon this fact will arise the important question, Can we prolong life?

CHAPTER II.

THE SOURCE OF THE ACCUMULATIONS WHICH CAUSE "OLD AGE" AND "NATURAL DEATH."

WE will now inquire into the *source* of these depositions, which gradually accumulate from the first period of existence to old age. Firstly, we will ask the source of the fibrinous and gelatinous substances; secondly, the source of the earthy deposits.

Oxygen is the most abundant of the elements; it forms eight-ninths of water, nearly one-fourth of the air, and about one-half of the chief constituents of the earth's surface.

In the air it exists, in combination chiefly with nitrogen, in the proportions as under:

Oxygen . . .	22
Nitrogen . .	78
	100

In a free state, *nitrogen* is comparatively *inactive*, but *oxygen*, although constituting only a comparatively small proportion of the atmosphere, is the *active* element.

Oxygen combines with all the known elements, with the exception of fluorine, forming oxides. Of that which is chemical in the animal economy, oxygen has perhaps the most important action, whether it be directly chemical, or chemical agency in action and reaction.

During respiration by the lungs, animals inhale the oxygen of the air, and expire or breathe out carbonic acid gas.

A middle-sized man consumes a little over 40,000 cubic inches of oxygen per day, by respiration. This oxygen being positive electricity, creates, or generates, a nitro-hydrogen, or negative action, at the skin and external surfaces. The lungs, heart, and vessels of the arterial system have therefore a positive action, whilst the skin, veins, and liver have a correlative, or negative action. This is chemical agency in action and reaction.

During life, every being throughout animated nature is in a constant state of change—waste by oxygen, renewal by food. The arteries, we may say, distribute oxygen universally, as a cause of the waste, whilst the veins absorb nitrogen, carbon, etc., as the products of that waste, thus giving rise to the union of oxygen with carbon, and to the expiration of carbonic acid gas.

The expiration of carbonic acid is therefore due to oxidation, or waste, of the substances of the body, which oxidation, together with that of the constituents of food, is the supposed source of animal heat.

The experiments of Regnault, Reiset, and Magnus,

prove that the lungs are not the seat of the *formation* of carbonic acid, but that carbonic acid is expelled from the blood in the lungs, and that oxygen is taken up in its place—that is, that a current of oxygen is conveyed throughout the system in the arterial blood, which in its passage causes waste, or oxidation, in the capillaries, and thus gives rise to the presence of carbonic acid in venous blood.

Atmospheric air in contact with the lungs undergoes a change; its nitrogen is returned free, together with the carbonic acid expelled from the blood, and part of the *oxygen*, taking the place of the carbonic acid, is carried onward in the arterial blood—now changed from the dark purple-red of venous blood to a bright red colour, by the loss of carbonic acid from the blood corpuscles, and their absorption of oxygen —to take part in many of the vital functions and numerous changes in the animal economy, which are so intimately connected with the new and acquired properties of arterial blood.

There are two substances existing in blood— *albumen* and *fibrin*. The following are their component elements:

	Albumen.	Fibrin.
Carbon	53.5	52.7
Hydrogen	7.0	6.9
Nitrogen	15.5	15.4
Oxygen	22.0	23.5
Sulphur	1.6	1.2
Phosphorus	0.4	0.3
	100.0	100.0

From this analysis we see that fibrin contains 1·5 per cent. more oxygen than albumen.

If we make a clear and strained solution of albumen, or white of egg, and place it in a vessel under circumstances which will not allow the admission of atmospheric air, and pass oxygen through it daily for from four to seven days, a whitish film, insoluble in cold water, is found floating on the surface. This substance is analogous in appearance and properties to the fibrin of blood.

Thus we may justly infer that fibrin, to use a general term, is an oxide of albumen.

The lacteals absorb the nutrient part of the products of digestion, the *azotised* substances of which exist either in an albuminous or minutely subdivided state,[*] and from *some cause* fibrin gradually increases in the contents of the absorbent system during its passage from the lacteals to the thoracic duct, from whence it passes into the blood.

"The proportion of fibrin has been supposed to increase as the *lymph* approaches the thoracic duct; thus from the *lumbar* lymphatics of a fasting horse, Gmelin obtained 0·25 per cent. of dry coagulum, and from that of the *thoracic duct* of the same animal, 0·42 per cent."—QUAIN.

[*] It has been proved by Majendie, Liebig, and others, that gelatine possesses no nutritive value. In the digestion of fibrin, as in its decomposition, "the putrefaction of a small portion causes the solution of the remainder." A certain portion of the fibrine during digestion is decomposed, the remainder gives up part of its oxygen to the decomposition, and becomes true albumen, coagulable by heat.

"The *chyle*, when taken from the *lacteal vessels*, before they have reached the glands, is generally found to coagulate less firmly than in the more advanced stage of the process."—*Ibid.*

In Dr. Carpenter's *Human Physiology*, the following relative proportions of fibrin in different parts of the absorbent system are given:

In the afferent or peripheral lacteals (from the intestines to the mesenteric glands)	Fibrin, *little*, or none.
In the efferent or central lacteals (from the mesenteric glands to the thoracic duct)	Fibrin, *medium* quantity.
In the thoracic duct	Fibrin, *maximum* quantity.

Thus from *some cause* fibrin increases in the absorbent system, and as we have shown that oxygen will convert albumen (which exists in the lacteals) into fibrin, we may justly infer that oxygen is the *cause* of this increase.

Precisely the same process of oxidation goes on in the blood, which contains about seven per cent. of albumen; this is gradually oxidised in the lungs and vessels, and converted into fibrin.

If we partially suspend the respiratory functions, therefore the process of oxidation in the lungs, the amount of fibrin is decreased in the blood, or, more correctly speaking, it is not formed to the same extent.

M. Dupuy found that "when the pneumogastric nerves were divided in the cervical region in horses, the quantity of fibrin in the blood became progressively diminished to a very remarkable extent."

Albuminous substances are being almost continually absorbed by the lacteals and poured into the blood; thus the supply is kept up, to be little by little converted into fibrin, which is kept in solution in the blood, so long as a certain amount of heat exists, and motion or circulation is given to it. This motion is decreased during circulation through the capillaries. Although much of the fibrin either oozes through their walls, and is deposited to nourish organs and structures and repair their waste, much of it accumulates, lessening the calibre of vessels, and indurating organs and structures. This accumulation is small, the blood usually containing only about three per cent of fibrin, but it is gradual and constant.

In old age, as well as fibrin, a large quantity of *gelatin* has accumulated.

Gelatin is never found in vegetables, *nor does it exist in the blood*, but it is found in the animal economy, in which it must therefore be *formed*.*

Its composition is—carbon, 50; hydrogen, 7;

---

* In the egg we see an instance of this transformation; albumen exists, what little fibrin there is being confined to the membranes, but there is *no gelatin*. In the *chick*, on hatching (a process which may be accomplished artificially, by the simple presence of heat, moisture, and atmospheric air), the amount of fibrin is found to have increased, and gelatin is found in comparatively large quantities. In the egg the former was found in minute quantities, the latter not at all. Where do they come from? Nothing has entered the egg from without but moisture and air containing *oxygen*. The action of oxygen on albumen is the cause.

THE SOURCE OF "OLD AGE."

nitrogen, 18; oxygen, 25. It therefore contains 1·5 per cent. more oxygen than fibrin. As fibrin is an oxide of albumen, so is gelatine an oxide of fibrin, and the large quantities existing in old age are due to the action of atmospheric *oxygen* on fibrin deposited from the blood. If we carry the process of oxidation still further, we find that part of these fibrinous and gelatinous substances are decomposed as the waste of tissues, and resolved into the compounds of ammonia and urea, and eliminated from the system;* but at the same time the gradual process of accumulation is going on; it is a battle between accumulation and removal. The former is the victor and gains the upper hand; hence the accumulation is greater than the elimination.

Thus the *fibrinous* and *gelatinous* accumulations found in old age are *caused by* the action of that never-resting, active, corroding, and destroying element, atmospheric *oxygen*.

The *earthy salts*, which we have already pointed out increase with age, are found by experiment to exist in different proportions in different individuals of the same age, which leads us to the conclusion

---

* "If ten eqs. of oxygen be added to albumen, a formula will be given containing the elements of the membranes and choleic acid."
—LIEBIG.

Further, that when uric acid is formed from gelatin, the elements of choleic acid (an important acid of the bile) remain, and we are of opinion that, at no late period, the formation of many of the complex constituents of the urine and bile, from substances originating from albumen, by the presence of a certain amount of heat, and by the simple additions of water and oxygen, will be demonstrably correct.

that these depositions arise from various causes, or, if from the same cause, variable in intensity. On the inner surface of an ordinary tea-kettle, after being regularly used for several months, a considerable amount of incrustation has taken place; and although it is generally believed that this incrustation arises from the deposition of earthy substances from the water, consequent upon boiling,* and rendering *insoluble* the previously *soluble* salts of lime, experiment shows that the great bulk of this incrustation arises from matter previously soluble being precipitated, in consequence of the water which held it in solution being driven off in the form of steam, and the water remaining in the vessel being thus more than saturated, the excess is thrown down.

Here we have a condition precisely similar to that which exists in the living human body, as the process of transpiration. Transpiration is nothing more or less than the evaporation and elimination of the fluids and gases of the system.

The basis of animal fluids is water, and these fluids

* The general impression is that *hard* water is caused by the presence of carbonate of lime held in solution by an excess of carbonic acid gas, and that on boiling the latter is eliminated, and the carbonate, being no longer soluble, is precipitated. This is, however, an error. Carbonates are not the cause of hard water, which state is due to the presence of sulphate of lime, or soluble gypsum. Thus, on washing with soap in hard water, a chemical decomposition takes place; the sulphuric acid of the sulphate of lime unites with the soda of the soap, forming sulphate of soda, which remains in solution, whilst the lime unites with the tallow, forming oleate and stereate of calcium, an insoluble compound which floats on the surface of the water.

hold certain compounds of lime in solution; and when, by transpiration, the watery basis is eliminated (precisely as in the common tea-kettle), a portion of these lime compounds is, and must be, deposited. And although much of the matter deposited is carried off in the *excretæ*, much also is left behind in the different organs and structures of the body, which, little by little increasing, forms accumulations which bring the individual to that stage of "old age" and decrepitude which terminates in "natural death."

In the lungs, "the air-tubes, after repeated divisions and sub-divisions, terminate in small vesicular cells, on the walls of which a minute capillary network of bloodvessels is distributed. The membrane which constitutes these cells, and through which the atmosphere acts upon the blood, is believed to be at least *thirty times* as extensive as the surface of the body. The lungs, therefore, constitute one vast *excreting* surface, from which is constantly escaping into the air a mixed *cloud* of carbonic acid gas and *water*."— HOOPER'S *Physician's Vade Mecum*.

The quantity of water exhaled from the lungs, according to the average estimates of different authorities, amounts to from seven ounces to one pint eleven ounces in the twenty-four hours.

Thus the lungs eliminate carbonic acid gas, water, and other *volatile* substances. *Earthy salts* are not volatile, and are therefore *not eliminated by the lungs*.

The *skin* eliminates chiefly *water* and carbonic

acid, also nitrogen, lactate and acetate of ammonia, and a *small quantity* of alkaline and *earthy salts*.

"It is calculated that about *three pounds of water* are daily conveyed to the surface as insensible perspiration." This is, however, increased during hot weather and by exercise.

The purpose of the *urine* is to remove a portion of the liquid and solid matters which have been taken into the system as food, also to carry off materials resulting from the waste or disorganisation of tissues. It is secreted by the kidneys from arterial blood, and contains in the thousand parts, on an average, nine hundred and fifty of water, the remaining fifty parts being composed of *organic* constituents—urea, uric, lithic, hippuric, and lactic acids; salts of ammonia and extractive matters; and *inorganic* constituents—carbonic, sulphuric, hydrochloric, and phosphoric acids, combined with soda, potash, magnesia, and lime. If we remove the water and collect one thousand parts of the solid matters, they are found to contain, on an average, sixteen parts, or 1·6 per cent., of *earthy* salts. Lehman's analysis gives 1·5 per cent.

The *solids* discharged in the urine in twenty-four hours average less than one and a half ounces; taking this, however, as an average, about twenty-one grains of earthy salts are daily eliminated by the kidneys; but a portion of the phosphates in the urine is secreted in the mucus of the bladder.

The amount of earthy salts in fæces excreted in the twenty-four hours is generally about one-fourth of the quantity voided in the urine, or a little more than five grains,* a small quantity of which is perhaps derived from the saliva and other secretions of digestion, the rest from articles taken into the system as diet, and on which the amount depends.

Owing to the many different conditions of quantity and quality of foods, hard and soft water, excretion by the skin and kidneys being increased by activity and hard work, and decreased inversely, thus varying in the amount of solid constituents according to the specific gravity of the urine, which alters slightly even hourly, it is impossible to collect a correct average of the amount of earthy salts taken into the system, and the amount excreted by it, from the many different authors, or even to obtain the same by *occasional* observation. We therefore determined to experiment on ourselves, by carefully weighing the amount of solids, and measuring the amount of liquids consumed, and calculating as minutely as possible, from the observations of well-authenticated analysts, and from our own made at the time, the amount of earthy matter they contained—*i.e.*, the amount taken into the system; and also by analysing and weighing the amount of earthy compounds carried off by the different excretæ. To avoid error, these experiments were carried on for some weeks, and always gave the same result: that *the amount taken into the system was greater than the amount*

* This item varies considerably, and is frequently very much larger.

eliminated.* This amount fluctuated daily, sometimes amounting to mere traces in the twenty-four hours. But if we multiply even traces by days and years, we find a considerable amount of earthy salts unaccounted for. We have already shown that they exist in larger quantities in the body in old age than in middle life, and in the latter than in childhood. They *are*, therefore, *retained and deposited in the system*, and, little by little increasing, give rise to the changes observed as age advances.

On removing the water from blood, and incinerating its solid constituents, 1·25 to 1·5 per cent. of ash is left. This is composed of hydrochlorate of soda and potash, carbonates and phosphates of soda, sulphate of potash, *phosphate of lime and magnesia, carbonates of lime and magnesia*, and peroxide of iron.

According to the analysis of M. Le Canu, for which he gained the prize given by the Académie Royale de Médecine of Paris, the compounds of lime, magnesia, and iron constitute 2·1 in the thousand parts of liquid human blood.

Thus in blood are certain proportions of calcareous matter.

As the *blood* is built up from the *chyle* (which is formed from the chyme by the action of the bile and pancreatic fluid), we should expect to find in the latter the same calcareous matter; *and such is the fact*, that, on analysis, we find the same earthy salts in the chyle as exist in the blood.

* The experiments of Boussingault, on horses, confirm this in animals.

As the *chyle* is formed from the *chyme* (which is the product of the action of the stomach and its secretions on food), we should in it find the same calcareous matter; and such, again, is the *fact*.

But as the *chyme* is the product of *digestion*, we expect to find the same calcareous matter in the contents of the stomach; and such also is the *fact*.

The contents of the stomach consist of food and drink taken to nourish and support the system, and in that food and drink we ought to find the same calcareous substances; and chemical analysis gives to us the certain answer, that the food and drink taken to support the system contain, besides the elements of nutrition, *earthy salts*, which are the *cause* of ossification, obstruction, old age, and natural death.

We have now traced these earthy compounds which are found in the system, and which increase as age advances, to the blood, from which they are, by the process of transpiration, gradually deposited. From the blood we trace them to the chyle, from the chyle to the chyme, and from the chyme to the contents of the stomach, and thence to articles of diet.

Thus we eat to live, and eat to die.*

As we have traced these earthy salts to our food or articles of diet, we naturally inquire whether the

* "In food we are constantly introducing different substances. which produce variations in the nutrition of the parts. These differences *accumulate* their influence in those changes named age, and they culminate in the final change named death."—G. H. LEWES, *Physiology of Common Life*.

different kinds of food and drink, which we have for our selection, contain the same proportion of ossifying and "old age" producing matter? Here chemical analysis answers in the negative! Some of the most generally used alimentary substances contain a comparatively *large* proportion of earthy compounds, some a *moderate*, and others a very *small* amount.

"No matter what kind of food we eat, or what fluid we drink, the earthy salts contained therein have all the same source—the earth."

If we eat vegetable food, plants derive their earthy salts from the earth in which they grow. If animal flesh be our sustenance, they have the same source, through the medium of the animal we eat, which derives its supply from vegetation.

Fish in the sea, fowl in the air, animals upon the earth, all derive the earthy salts contained in them originally from the earth, in the food on which they live.

Any organ, or all the organs put together, of man or any being, cannot *generate* any element; hence *all that is earthy in man is derived from the earth.*

From this it follows, that if we can so regulate our diet—food and drink—that the amount of earthy matter taken into the system be sufficient only for the growth and nourishment of the bones, without which our powers of strength and motion would be useless (the body being deprived of its mechanical levers), the many organs and structures would not, and could not, harden and ossify; the arteries would not become indurate and lessened in calibre, capillaries would not become obliterated, the brain would not decrease in size by age, sight would not fail, hearing, taste, and smell would not lose their susceptibility, hair would not turn grey, the skin would not become dry and wrinkled, the body would retain its fluidity, elasticity, and activity, and the brain its mental capabilities.

If we can so regulate our diet that these earthy compounds are taken into the system in *smaller* quantities, and therefore take a *longer* period to accumulate—if we can even partially accomplish this—we can prolong life.

We have shown "old age" and "natural death" to be due to two causes—*firstly*, to the action of atmospheric *oxygen*, which consumes our bodies and causes fibrinous and gelatinous accumulations; *secondly*, to a deposition of earthy matter (ossification). If, therefore, we can, by artificial means, partially arrest the never-ceasing action of atmospheric oxygen, and at the same time prevent the accumulations of these earthy compounds, or even remove them from the system—that state of body termed "old age" would be deferred, and life would be prolonged for a *lengthened period.*

* * * * * *

"Many of the fundamental or leading ideas of the present time appear, to him who knows not what science has already achieved, as extravagant as the notions of the alchemists."—LIEBIG.

* * * * * *

In all the animal kingdom there is a beauty of structure manifested, wondrous, marvellous, and exquisite; but man *alone* has been endowed with knowledge, wisdom, and understanding, as a sole and exclusive gift to him.

Speaking of the patriarchs, Josephus affirms: "*Their food was fitter for the prolongation of life;* and besides, God afforded them a longer time of life on account of their virtue, and the good use they made of it in astronomical and geometrical discoveries."

Many authors contend that the years, at the time of the patriarchs, were shorter than the present time —not more than one-fourth the period. If this were true, Methusaleh would have lived only two hundred and forty-three years, Terah fifty-one, and Abram forty-four. Enoch would have been only sixteen when he begat Methusaleh, Arphaxad eight and three-quarters when he begat Salah, Salah seven years old when he begat Eber, and Adam would have been more than a great grandfather at thirty-three. There is no evidence to show the years were less than at the present time. It is probable, and quite possible (presuming that their diet tended to longevity), that the patriarchs lived to their recorded ages.*

---

* The extraordinary longevity of the patriarchs may be traced [1] to their diet, which consisted firstly of fruits, afterwards to a great extent of the flesh of young and tender animals,—the calf, the kid, and the lamb. The flesh of young animals contain an excess of phosphoric acid, which prevents lime accumulating in the system ; from this cause alone, great longevity would result. [2.] There was a less percentage

Who, therefore, can deny, that with all our knowledge and discoveries, which are daily increasing, man may not again re-discover the secret of long life, which has been lost for so many ages, and which secret may probably be summed up in the following few words : If a human being subsists upon food which contains a large proportion of lime, a large proportion will

of oxygen in the air. They wasted less than we do now, therefore they required less food. Europeans and Americans at the present time eat from three to five meals a day; the patriarchs of old did not. They had one good meal occasionally; young flesh was its chief constituent, and it often took more than a day to prepare. [3] The surface soil contained more potash and less lime than now, consequently the herbs, or animals feeding on them, contained less of the latter, and were better adapted to longevity.

The record of the ages of the Patriarchs coincides exactly with what science is able to trace. From Adam and Methusaleh, who are stated to have lived over nine hundred years, the longevity gradually decreases a few years, less and less, with considerable regularity, until we come to Joseph, who lived little over a hundred years. The ages when children were born unto them decrease with the same regularity. The earlier patriarchs were about 100 years old, the latter thirty or less when they begat children. Development was slower at first, but as the above circumstances altered, maturity was arrived at in less time, and the period of life decreased in the same ratio.—*Original Eden*, by the Author.

Scientists, or otherwise, who dispute or deny the Mosaic records of the early patriarchs, remind us of a rich coal merchant, we knew some years ago. We drew diagrams of the *Lepido-dendron sigillaria* and other carboniferous plants, to explain to him the origin of coal. His remarks were, "I've sold more coals than any one I knows. What I say is, Coals *is* coals, and always *was* coals!" Those who deny patriarchal longevity, are in the same amusing position. They know what *is*, they have not the knowledge, nor have they taken the trouble, to ascertain what *was!*

The patriarchs of old, according to Josephus, knew that the *great year* was accomplished only after the lapse of 600 years.

M. Cassini, of the Paris Observatory, says, "This period (the enter into the composition of the chyme, the chyle, and the blood; and as from the blood the deposition of lime takes place, the greater the amount of lime that blood contains, the greater will be the amount deposited in the system, the greater the degree of ossification, and the sooner will be produced that rigidity, inactivity, and decrepitude, which makes him old and brings him to *premature death*.

On the other hand, if the food and drink taken to nourish and support the body are selected from the articles which contain the *least* amount of lime, the least amount will enter into the composition of the chyme, the chyle, and the blood, the less amount will there be to deposit, the less the degree of ossification, the less the rigidity, inactivity, and decrepitude, and the *longer the life of the man* !

great cycle of 600 years) is one of the most remarkable that has been discovered; for if we take the lunar month to be 29 days, 12 hours, 44 minutes, 3 seconds, we find that 219,146¼ days make 7,421 lunar months, and that this number of days gives 600 solar years of 365 days, 5 hours, 51 minutes, 36 seconds. If this was in use before the Deluge, it appears very probable, it must be confessed, that the patriarchs were already acquainted to a considerable degree of accuracy with the motion of the stars, for *this lunar month agrees to a second, almost, with that which has been determined by modern astronomers.*"
—FLAMMARION."

CHAPTER III.

DIET IN COMPOSITION AND QUANTITY AS BEST ADAPTED TO A PROLONGED EXISTENCE.

BEFORE entering directly upon the subject of diet and its composition, we venture a few remarks upon the structure and organisation of man, relative to his adapation for a prolonged existence.

If we view the genus *Homo*, either as a whole or in its division, irrespective of colour, climate, or habit, we find a great similarity in both an anatomical and a physiological sense. The structure, organisation, and functions are the same in one and all. The body of man is perfect, its Creator "saw that it was good"; the same Creator gave to man wisdom, and it is a duty to that Creator to use such wisdom in gaining knowledge which will enable him to keep that body perfect.

"Like the pious pilgrim to the Holy Land, toil on in search of the sacred shrine, in search of truth—God's truth, God's laws—as manifested in His works, in His creation."—H.R.H. THE LATE PRINCE CONSORT.

"The human body, as a machine, is perfect . . . it

is apparently intended to go on for ever."—DR. MUNRO.

"If we could imagine a physiologist seeing for the first time an organised structure, such as the human frame, in a state of perfection, however closely he might examine it, and however intimately he might know the structure, he could not, without the knowledge of experience, pretend to say there appeared any reason why death should occur; he could not, indeed, conceive such a thought as death."—DR. REDFORD.

"Such a machine as the human frame, unless accidentally depraved, or injured by some external cause, would seemed formed for perpetuity."—*Medical Conspectus*, DR. GREGORY.

"If a living organised being be examined at the epoch of its greatest perfection . . . a mutuality of cause and effect is perceived which almost promises immortality."—SIR T. C. MORGAN.

"At some future day there can be little doubt that the value and duration of life will be *extended* greatly beyond what it is at present—*greatly beyond*, perhaps, *what we at present can imagine.*"—*Medical Dictionary*, by DR. THOMSON.

"If the repair were always identical with the waste, never varying in the slightest degree, life would then only be terminated by some accident, *never by old age.*"—*The Physiology of Common Life*, by G. H. LEWES.

The body is in a constant state of change—of waste

and renewal. Oxygen consumes and wastes the many different tissues; we take food to supply the loss; in that food we take into the system the elements of destruction—earthy salts. As we have already stated, every organ and structure, up to a certain period of life, has the power of reproducing and repairing any waste, after which period the blood-vessels become so indurated and lessened in calibre, that the powers of irrigating and nourishing the various structures decline. Could these channels be kept free from any obstruction, the brain would act, because the heart would act; the heart would act, because the brain would act as a perpetual motion; the functions would maintain the organisation; the renewal would be equal to the waste and decay; there would be a harmony and mutuality of cause and effect; and man, could this be effected, would have an existence almost *promising immortality*.

We are not justified in putting a *limit* to the days of man; science fails to prove one, religion does not dictate one. The well-known expression, " The days of our years are threescore years and ten," is *not* an *edict* from God, but simply a *lamentation* that the term of life was so reduced by the wickedness and ignorance of the people.

Were it not for the superstitions, prejudices, and tyrannies which kept humanity, as it were, underground; were it not for the theories and hypotheses which are made to explain phenomena before their cause is known; our knowledge would be of a more rational, purer, and more complete kind; one branch of science would not be constantly waging war against another; the investigations and discoveries of to-day would have no need of contradiction to-morrow; all would be harmony and progression.

Facts, designs, and discoveries, which have been for a time neglected, despised, or ridiculed, one by one arise to reproach ignorance and benefit humanity. These are generally the result of investigation, which we are not on any grounds justified in arresting.

"It is perfectly vain to attempt to stop investigation. . . . Depend upon it, if a chemist, by bringing the proper materials together, could produce a human body, he would do it. And why not? There is no command forbidding him to do it; his inquiries are limited solely by his own capacity."—PROF. TYNDAL.

We are justified in carrying our investigations, if they are for the benefit of man, in either mind, body, or estate, to the utmost limit, in the firm belief and under the true conviction, that "The effort to extend the dominion of man over nature is the most healthy and most noble of all ambitions."—BACON.

When we view the majority of mankind in relation to his diet, our knowledge of his habits and disposition points out to us the many difficulties to be surmounted in ordering any alteration in his predisposed and acquired indulgences; indeed, the difficulties are so great, that we are induced to quote the following:

DIET AND PROLONGED EXISTENCE. 73

"The common definition of man is false; he is not a reasoning animal. The best you can predict of him is, that he is an animal *capable* of reasoning."—WARBURTON.

This is true in many cases; it is very true in regard to his diet. And further, as Cato observes, "It is a hard and difficult task to undertake to dispute with men's stomachs, which have no ears."

Some men have, perhaps, no cares, others pass an existence which may be a constant scene of trouble; but how many of these think there is no other pleasure in life but in eating, drinking, and sleeping! Many men at a certain age become lost to the other enjoyments of life, and these become the only pleasures they recognise. This wonderful being of creation, whose place is to have dominion over all things, dies—true, he has lived, but in *many* cases he has done no good to himself; he has not benefited those around him, or those that come after him. Yet he *has lived*, and expects to be rewarded with a seat in heaven. For what?

Surely there is a better purpose in man's existence than mere eating, drinking, and sleeping, resembling the life of the lower animals. Man has a higher destiny and a nobler purpose; he should aim to give happiness to himself and those around him. He is lord of creation; let him strive to become its ruler and benefactor.

Many men are ruled and governed by their diet— their "belly is their God." Many undertakings are influenced by the same, whether they be the meeting of relations and friends for pleasure or for pain, for marriage or the funeral, commercial transactions, the meetings of lodges, clubs, or guilds; societies with the banner of "Charity" unfurled above them, whether they be ecclesiastical, constitutional, or benevolent; meetings for social, agricultural, scientific, judicial, and political purposes; congresses for peace or war—for the destruction or preservation of men; all these different assemblies meet in a social and friendly manner. The banquet has become an institution; even Her Majesty's ministers have "YE ANNUALE WHYTEBAITE DINNER, for ye sadde and sobere comforte of frendes, and ye guestes are bydden to eate after ye *Hungarie* mannere."

How many diseases can be traced to over-eating! How few to moderation or eating little! When will man, who is *capable* of reasoning, use that reason? When will he remove the mist from his eyes, which has shrouded them for so many generations?

When he does this he will see that the *object* of his diet is to keep up a balance between waste and renewal —to give an *equilibrium* to the system.

BEANS (*Faba vulgaris*).

Water	14·8
Caseine	24·0
Starch	36·0
Sugar	2·0
Gum	8·5
Fat	2·5
Woody fibre	9.2
Mineral matter (ashes)	3·5
Total	100·0

DIET AND PROLONGED EXISTENCE.

BARLEY (*Hordeum distichum*).

Water	14.0
Gluten	12.8
Albumen	0.0*
Starch	48.0
Sugar	3.8
Gum	3.7
Fat	0.3
Fibre	13.2
Ashes	4.2
Total	100.0

ASH OF BARLEY.

Silica	29.67
Phosphoric acid	36.80
Sulphuric acid	0.16
Chlorine	0.15
Peroxide of iron	0.83
Lime	3.23
Magnesia	4.30
Potash	16.00
Soda	8.86
Total	100.00

EINHOFF.

OATS (*Avena sativa*).

"The outer husk of oats, unlike wheat, is poor in flesh-formers, so that oatmeal is better than the whole oat as food. In making oatmeal, one quarter of oats (328 lbs.) yields 188 lbs. of meal and 74 lbs. of husks, the rest being water. Oatmeal is remarkable for its large amount of fat."

Water	13.6
Flesh-formers (gluten, albumen, etc.)	17.0†
Starch	39.7

* Einhoff gives albumen in barley as 1.15 in 100 parts.

† Sibson found gluten in oats to the extent of 11.85 in 100; in oatmeal, 15.68 in 100. Vogel gives 4 parts of albumen in 100 of oatmeal.

Sugar	5·4
Gum	3·0
Fat	5·7
Fibre	12·6
Mineral matters (ashes)	3·0
Total	**100·0**

RYE (*Secale cereale*).

Water	13·00
Gluten	10·79
Albumen	3·04
Starch	51·14
Gum	5·31
Sugar	3·74
Fat	0·95
Woody fibre	10·29
Mineral matter (ashes)	1·74
Total	**100·00**

ULTIMATE ANALYSIS OF WHEAT, RYE, AND OATS, DRIED AT 230° F.

	Wheat	Rye.	Oats.
Carbon	46·1	46·2	50·7
Hydrogen	5·8	5·6	6·4
Oxygen	43·4	44·2	36·7
Nitrogen	2.3	1·7	2·2
Ashes	2·4	2·3	4·0
Total	**100·0**	**100·0**	**100·0**

BOUSSINGAULT.

MAIZE, OR INDIAN CORN (*Zea Mays*).

Water	14·0
Gluten	12·0
Albumen	0·0*
Starch	60·0
Sugar and Gum	0·3
Fat	7·7
Fibre	5·0
Mineral Matter (ashes)	1·0
Total	**100·0**

* Brande gives albumen 2.5; Graham gives the same quantity.

RICE (*Orysa sativa*).

Water	13.5
Gluten	6.5
Starch	74.1
Sugar	0.4
Gum	1.0
Fat	0.7
Fibre	3.3
Mineral matter (ashes)	0.5
Total	**100.0**

MALT.

Starch	69.0
Gum	14.0
Sugar	16.0
Gluten	1.0
Total	**100.0**

Dr. Thompson.

PEAS (*Pisum sativum*).

Water	14.1
Caseine	23.4
Starch	37.0
Sugar	2.0
Gum	9.0
Fat	2.0
Woody fibre	10.0
Mineral ashes	2.5
Total	**100.0**

Dr. Pereira gives:

Starch	32.45
Amylaceous fibre	21.88
Legumine (caseine)	14.56
Gum	6.37
Albumen	1.72
Sweet extractive	2.11
Water	14.06
Salts (ashes)	6.56
Loss	.29
Total	**100.00**

GARDEN BEANS (*Vicia faba*).

Starch	34·17
Amylaceous fibre	15·89
Legumine (caseine)	10·86
Gum	4·61
Albumen	0·81
Sweet extractive matter	3·54
Membrane	10·05
Water	15·63
Salts (ashes)	3·46
Loss	0·98
Total	100·00

EINHOFF.

KIDNEY BEAN (*Phaseolus vulgaris*).

Starch	35·94
Amylaceous fibre	11·07
Legumine (caseine)	20·81
Gum	19·37
Albumen	1·35
Sweet extractive	3·41
Membrane	7·50
Water	(dried)
Salts (ashes)	0·55
Total	100·00

EINHOFF.

LENTILS (*Ervum lens*).

"Lentils, like other leguminous seeds, contain much caseine. They are a favourite food in the East. The Hindoo adds lentils to his starch-giving rice, and obtain from them the nourishment the latter does not contain . . . Lentils are particularly nutritious. . . . The food sold under the name of 'Revalenta Arabica' is the meal of the lentil after being freed from its outer skin, which is indigestible The 'red pottage' for which Esau sold his birthright appears to have been made of lentils. One hundred parts contain, so far as is known:"

Water	14·0
Caseine	26·0
Starch	35·0
Sugar	2·0
Gum	7·0
Fat	2·0
Woody fibre	12·5
Mineral matter	1·5
Total	100·0

According to Dr. Pereira, lentils consist of:

Starch	32·81
Amylaceous fibre.	18·75
Legumine (caseine)	37·32
Gum	5·99
Albumen	1·15
Sweet extractive	3·12
Water	(dried)?
Salts	0·57
Loss	0·29
Total	100·00

BUCKWHEAT (*Polyponum fagopyrum*).

"Buckwheat is known in this country by the name of 'brank,' and is cultivated for the sake of its green fodder. It is sometimes mixed with wheat-flour. Birds are exceedingly fond of it, and one of the principal uses made of it in this country is to feed pheasants in the winter."

It consists of:

Water	14·2
Gluten	8·6
Starch	50·0
Gum	2·0
Sugar	2·0
Fat	1·0
Woody fibre	20·4
Mineral matter (ashes)	1·8
Total	100·0

VEGETABLE ROOTS.

Potato (*Solanum tuberosum*).

Water	75·2
Flesh-formers (albumen, gluten, etc.)	1·4
Starch	15·5
Dextrine	0·4
Sugar	3·2
Fat	0·2
Fibre	3·2
Ashes	0·9
Total	100·0

According to Einhoff, the potato contains:

Albumen and mucilage	5·4
Starchy matter	22·0
Water, salts, and loss	72·6
Total	100·0

Dr. Pereira gives:

Water	66·875
Starch and amylaceous fibre	30·469
Albumen	0·503
Gluten	0·055
Fat	0·056
Gum	0·020
Asparagin	0·063
Extractive	0·921
Chloride of potassium	0·176
Silicate, phosphate, and citrate of iron, manganese, alumina, soda, potash and lime	0·815
Free citric acid	0·047
Total	100·000

Parsnips (*Pastinaca sativa*).

Water	82·039
Albumen and caseine	1·215
Sugar	2·882

Starch	3·507
Fat	0·546
Gum	0·748
Woody fibre	8·022
Ashes	1·041
Total	**100·000**

TURNIPS (*Brassica rapa*).

Water	90·5
Albumen and caseine	1·1
Sugar	4·0
Gum	1·5
Woody fibre	2·4
Mineral matter (ashes)	0·5
Total	**100·0**

According to Dr. Pereira, the turnip contains:

Water	92·5
Solid matter	7·5
Total	**100·0**

Ultimate composition of dried turnips:

Carbon	42·9
Hydrogen	5·5
Oxygen	42·3
Nitrogen	1·7
Ashes	7·6
Total	**100·0**

CARROTS (*Daucus carota*).

Water	87·5
Albumen and caseine	0·6
Sugar	6·4
Fat	0·2
Gum	1·0
Woody fibre	3·3
Mineral matter (ashes)	1·0
Total	**100·0**

The *Juice* of the carrot contains:

Fixed oil (some part volatile)	1·00
Red crystalline substance (carotin)	·34
Uncrystallisable sugar, with starch and malic acid	93·71
Albumen	4·35
Ashes (alumina, lime, iron)	·60
Total	100·00

PEREIRA.

SWEET POTATO (*Convolvulus Batatas*).

"The sweet potato is eaten largely in tropical America."

Water	57·50
Starch	16·05
Sugar	20·20
Albumen	1·50
Fat	0·30
Woody fibre	0·45
Gum, etc.	1·10
Ashes	2·90
Total	100·00

ONIONS.

Acrid volatile oil,
Uncrystallisable sugar,
Gum,
Vegetable albumen,
Woody fibre,
Acetic and phosphoric acids,
Phosphate and carbonate of lime,
Water.

PEREIRA.

According to Vaquelin and Fourcroy, the onion consists of: A white, acrid, volatile, and odorous oil; sulphur combined with oil, which makes it fœtid. A large quantity of uncrystallisable sugar; a large quantity of mucilage, like gum arabic; a vegeto-animal matter, coagulable by heat and analogous to gluten; phosphoric acid, *in part free*, in part combined with lime; acetic acid; citrate of lime; and a very tender fibrous matter, retaining some vegeto-animal matter.

"Garlic, leeks, and shalots have a similar composition."

OTHER VEGETABLES.

CABBAGE.

Extractive matter	2·34
Gummy extractive	2·89
Resin	0·05
Vegetable albumen	0·29
Fecula	0·63
Water, with acetic acid, sulphate and nitrate of potash, chloride of potassium, malate and phosphate of lime, phosphate of magnesia, iron, and manganese	93·80
Total	100·00

PEREIRA.

According to Sibson, the cabbage contains 1·87 per cent. of inorganic matter (ashes).

"The cabbage, dried, contains 30 to 35 per cent. of gluten."

CAULIFLOWER.

Colouring matter, mucilage, resin, vegetable albumen (about)	0·5
Chlorophylle, fatty matter, pectic acid (a product?) woody fibre (about)	1·8
Water, rather more than	90·0
Silica, malate of ammonia, malate of lime, *free* malic acid, acetate of potash, phosphate of lime, chloride of calcium, and sulphate of potash	traces

PEREIRA.

"Cauliflower, *dried*, contains gluten, sometimes as high as 64 per cent."

Asparagus consists of:
  Asparagine (asparamide),
  Gum,
  Uncrystallisable sugar,
  Vegetable albumen,
  Resin,
  Woody fibre,
  Acetate, malate, phosphate, and muriate of potash, lime, and iron.

CUCUMBER.

"The fresh peel contains solid matters similar to those of the peeled fruit, but containing much fungus-like matter 15·0, water 85·0, in 100·0.

Green and peeled, the cucumber consists of:

Sugar and extractive	1·66
Chlorophylle	0.04
Odorous matter	?
Fungus-line membrane	?
Soluble albumen	0·13
Phosphate of lime	0·53
Free phosphoric acid, an ammoniacal salt, malate, phosphate, sulphate, and muriate of potash, with sulphate of lime and iron	0·50
Water	97·14
Total	100·00

MUSHROOMS (*Morels*).

Stearine and elaine	4· 0
Sugar	2· 0
Albumen	1· 2
Azotised extract, or vegetable osmazome	29· 4
Fungine	39· 6
Gummy azotised extractive	5· 4
Boletate, and phosphate of ammonia and potash	8· 0
Water	10· 0
Total	98·16

BRANDE.

FRUITS.

DATES.

(The Flesh).

Uncrystallisable sugar	58·0
Pectine	8·9
Gum	3·4
Bassorine	4·1
Fatty matter	0·2
Wax	0·1
Fibre, with traces of colouring matter, and tannic acid	2·3
Water	23.0
Total	100·0

PEREIRA.

(The Kernel.)

Fibre	39·6
Gummy matter	36·4
Gum and mucus	2·5
Epidermis (albumen)	0·6
An astringent acid (catechu ?)	7·1
Stearine	0·5
Oleine	0·3
Water	13·0
Total	100·0

Ibid.

SWEET ALMONDS.

Fixed oil	54·0
Emulsin	24·0
Liquid sugar	6·0
Gum	3·0
Seed-coats	5·0
Woody fibre	4·0
Water	3·5
Acetic acid and loss	0·5
Total	100·0

Ibid.

BITTER ALMONDS.

Volatile oil and hydrocyanic acid, quantity undetermined	0·0
Fixed oil	28·0
Emulsin	30·0
Liquid sugar	6·5
Gum	3·0
Seed-coats	8·5
Woody fibre	5·0
Loss	19·0
Total	100·0

PEREIRA.

FIGS.

Granular sugar (glucose)	62·5
Fatty matter	0·9
Extractive, with chloride of calcium	0·4
Gum, with phosphoric acid	5·2
Woody fibre, and *achenia*	15·0
Water	16·0
Total	100·0

Ibid.

GRAPE (*Juice, when ripe*).

Extractive,
Sugar, granular and uncrystallisable,
Gum,
Glutinous matter
Malic acid (a little),
Citric acid (a little),
Tannic acid,
Bitartrate of potash,

Another analysis (*Juice when ripe*).

Odorous matter,
Sugar,
Gum,
Glutinous matter,
Malic acid and malate of lime,
Bitartrate of potash,
Supertartrate of lime.

(*Juice, when unripe*).

Wax,
Chlorophylle,
Tannin,
Glutinous matter (deposit from the juice),
Extractive,
Sugar (uncrystallisable)
Gallic acid,
Tartaric acid (free), about 1·12 per cent.
Mallic acid (free), about 2·19 per cent.
Bitartrate of potash,
Malate, phosphate, sulphate, and muriate of lime.

TAMARIND.

Citric acid	9·40
Tartaric acid	1·55
Malic acid	0·45
Bitartrate of potash	3·25
Sugar	12·50
Gum	4·70
Vegetable jelly, pectine	6·25
Parenchyma (liquorice)	34·35
Water	27·55
Total	100·00

PEREIRA.

ORANGE (*Juice*).

Citric acid,   Sugar,
Malic acid,   Citrate of lime,
Mucilage,   Water.
Albumen.

MELON (*Flesh*).

Crystallisable sugar	1·5
Pectic acid	traces
Uncrystallisable sugar, vegetable albumen, mucilage, free acid, saponifiable fat, nitrogenous matter, colouring matter, aromatic matter, starch, lignine, salts, water	98·5
Total	100·0

Ibid.

LEMON (*Juice*).

Citric acid, Bitter extractive,
Malic acid, Water.
Gum.

RED CURRANT (*Juice*).

Citric acid, Vegetable jelly,
Malic acid, Gum,
Sugar, Extractive.

PEREIRA.

BLACK CURRANT.

"Constituents similar to those of the red currant, with the addition of a peculiar volatile principle, and a violet colouring matter."

GOOSEBERRIES.

	Unripe.	Ripe.
Nitrogenous matter	1.07	0.86
Colouring mattter	0.03	0.00
Lignine and Seeds	8.45	8.01
Gum (Pectine?)	1.36	0.78
Sugar	0.52	6.24
Malic acid	1.80	2.41
Citric acid	0.12	0.31
Lime	0.24	0.29
Water	86.41	81.10
Total	100.00	100.00

Ibid.

MULBERRIES.

Colouring matter Sugar,
Pectine Woody fibre,
Bitartrate of potash, Water,

PINEAPPLE (*Juice*).

Peculiar aroma, Citric acid,
Sugar, Tartaric acid,
Gum, Water.
Malic acid,

RASPBERRY.

Volatile oil,
Citric acid,
Malic acid,
Crystallisable fermentable sugar,
Red colouring matter,
Mucus,
Woody fibre,
Pectine,
Ashes containing carbonate, phosphate, and muriate of potash, carbonate and phosphate of lime and magnesia; silica and oxide of iron.

STRAWBERRY.

Peculiar volatile aroma,
Sugar,
Mucilage,
Pectine,
Citric and malic acids, equal parts,
Woody fibre,
Pericarp, and water.

APRICOT.

	Unripe.	Ripe.
Nitrogenous matter	0.76	0.17
Colouring matter	0.04	0.10
Lignine	3.61	1.86
Gum (pectine?)	4.10	5.12
Sugar	traces	16.48
Malic acid	2.10	1.83
Lime, very small quantity	...	...
Water	89.39	74.44
Total	100.00	100.00

PEREIRA.

GREENGAGE.

	Unripe.	Ripe.
Nitrogenous matter	0.45	0.28
Colouring matter	0.03	0.08
Lignine	1.26	1.11
Gum (pectine?)	5.53	2.06
Sugar	17.71	24.81
Malic acid	0.45	0.56
Lime	trace	trace
Water	74.57	71.10
Total	100.00	100.00

Ibid.

In the analyses of the apricot, greengage, peach, and cherry, Dr. Pereira has omitted pectine, which is contained in most fruits. He remarks: "Pectine, or vegetable jelly, is here omitted, but is also contained in currants (red, white, and black), apples (both sweet and sour), pears, quinces, strawberries, bilberries, mulberries, cherries, love-apples, oranges, lemons, guava, tamarind, also in the Jerusalem artichoke and onion, in the carrot, turnip, celery, beet, etc."

PEACH.

	Unripe.	Ripe.
Nitrogenous matter	0·41	0·93
Colouring matter	0·27	0·00
Lignine	3·01	1·21
Gum (Pectine?)	4·22	4·85
Sugar	0·63	11·61
Malic acid	1·07	1·10
Lime	0·08	0·06
Water	90·31	80·24
Total	100·00	100·00

PEREIRA.

CHERRY.

	Unripe.	Ripe.
Nitrogenous matter	0·20	0·57
Colouring matter	0·05	0·00
Lignine	2·44	1·12
Gum (Pectine?)	6·01	3·23
Sugar	1·12	18·12
Malic acid	1·75	2·01
Lime	0·14	0·10
Water	88·29	74·85
Total	100·00	100·00

Ibid.

Pears (*Jargonelle*).

	Unripe.	Ripe.	Rotten.
Nitrogenous matter	0.08	0.21	0.301
Colouring matter	0.08	0.01	0.000
Resin, soluble in alcohol	0.00	0.00	0.058
Lignine	3.80	2.19	2.534
Gum (Pectine?)	3.17	2.07	3.400
Sugar	6.45	11.52	11.417
Malic acid	0.11	0.08	0.786
Lime	0.03	0.04	traces
Water	86.28	83.88	81.500
Total	100.00	100.00	99.996

Apples (*Average Composition*).

Nitrogenous matter	0.44
Colouring matter	0.10
Lignine	1.40
Gum	3.45
Sugar	16.50
Malic acid	1.10
Lime	0.01
Water	77.00
Total	100.00

ANIMAL FOOD.

100 parts of muscle or lean of

	Water.	Albumen or fibrine.	Gelatine.
Beef contains	74	20	6
Veal ,,	75	19	6

100 parts of muscle or lean of

	Water.	Albumen or fibrine.	Gelatine.
Mutton contains	71	22	7
Pork ,,	76	19	5
Chicken ,,	73	20	7
Codfish ,,	79	14	7
Haddock ,,	82	13	5
Sole ,,	79	15	6

BRANDE

Composition per cent. of carcases, excluding head and feet:

Animals as fattened for the butcher.	Mineral matter.	Dry nitrogenous substance.	Fat.	Total dry substance.	Water.
Calf	4.5	16.5	16.5	37.5	62.5
Bullock	5.0	15.0	30.0	50.0	50.0
Lamb	3.5	11.0	35.0	49.5	50.5
Sheep	3.5	12.5	40.0	56.0	44.0
Pig	1.5	10.0	50.0	61.5	38.5

Composition, in 100 parts:

	Mineral matter.	Gelatine.	Fibrine or albumen.	Fat.	Water.
Veal	4.5	7.5	9.0	16.5	62.5
Beef	5.0	7.0	8.0	30.0	50.0
Mutton	3.5	7.0	5.5	40.0	44.0
Pork	1.5	5.5	4.5	50.0	38.5

The following analysis by De Bibra gives a proximate idea of the *proportions* of alkaline and earthy salts in muscle:

Muscles dried at 100° C.	Percentage of Ashes in Muscles.	Alkaline Phosphate.	Phosphate of Lime.	Sea-Salt.	Sulphate of Soda.
Hare	4.48	79.80	15.10	4.20	0.90
Roebuck	4.68	72.00	20.60	1.00	...
Ox	7.71	76.80	16.40	6.50	...
Calf	...	89.80	10.20	...	...
Fowl	5.51	84.72	13.89	1.39	...
Wild-duck	4.48	84.00	14.80	1.20	...
Perch	7.08	54.39	44.34	1.27	...
Carp	6.10	44.19	42.20	1.31	12.30

Cheese (*Cheddar*).

Water	36·0
Curd, caseine, or cheesy matter	29·0
Fatty matter, or butter	30·5
Ashes (bone material)	6·5
Total	102·0

Cheese (*Skim-milk*).

Water	44·0
Curd, caseine, or cheesy matter	45·0
Fatty matter, or butter	6·0
Ashes	5·0
Total	100·0

SIBSON.

Milk (*Cow's*).

Water	86·0
Caseine	5·0
Butter	3·5
Sugar of milk	4·5
Salts	1·0
Total	100·0

Milk (*Ass's*).

Water	90·0
Caseine	2·0
Butter	1·5
Sugar of milk	6·0
Salts	0·5
Total	100·0

According to Berzelius, Milk contains:

Water	928·75
Curd, with a little cream	28·00
Sugar of milk	35·00
Muriate of potash	1·70
Phosphate of potash	0·25
Lactic acid and acetate of potash, with a trace of lactate of iron	6·00
Earthy phosphates	0·30
Total	1000·00

MILK (*Human*).

Water	89·5
Casein	3·0
Butter	3·0
Sugar of milk	4·0
Salts	0·5
Total	100·0

Earthy matter, obtained by incineration of 1,000 parts of cow's milk. Two instances:

	I.	II.
Phosphate of lime	2·31	3·44
Phosphate of magnesia	0·42	0·64
Phosphate of peroxide of iron	0·07	0·07
Total	2·80	4·15

HAIDLEN.

The total *ash* in these instances was 4·90 and 6·77 respectively; the earthy matter, therefore, amounted to more than half.

The flesh of most *fish* contains from 1·2 to 1·4 per cent. of salts, a less average than most animal foods.

COMPOSITION OF THE OYSTER.—PASQUIER.

Flesh.		*Liquor or Water.*
Fibrin	⎫	Osmazome
Albumen	⎪	Albumen
Gelatin	⎬ 12·16	Chloride of sodium
Osmazome	⎪	Sulphate of lime
Mucus	⎭	Sulphate of magnesia
Water	87·4	Chloride of magnesia
		Water
Total	100·0	

"By incineration, the organic matters yield 1·84 of a white ash, containing phosphate of lime, and the same salts as the liquor contains."

DIET AND PROLONGED EXISTENCE. 95

From analyses of foods, we see that fruits, as distinct from vegetables, have the least amount of earthy matter: most of them contain a large quantity of water, but that water in itself is of the purest kind—a distilled water of Nature, and has in solution vegetable albumen.

We also notice that they are to a great extent free from the *oxidised* albumens—glutinous and fibrinous substances, and many of them contain *acids*—citric, tartaric, malic, etc.—which, when taken into the system, act directly upon the blood, by increasing its solubility; by thinning it the process of circulation is more easily carried on, and the blood flows more easily in the capillaries (which become lessened in calibre as age advances) than it would if of a thicker nature. By this means the blood flows easily in vessels which have been perhaps for years lost to the passage of a thicker fluid. Further, these acids *lower* the temperature of the body, therefore the process of wasting, combustion, or oxidation, which increases in ratio to the temperature of the body, as indicated by the thermometer.

These acids are chiefly compounds of carbon, hydrogen, and oxygen; they differ from the mineral acids in being, as it were, burnt up in the system, and are therefore not traceable to the secretions and excretions.

Some fruits contain tannic acid, which acts beneficially on the system, by tanning or hardening the albuminous and gelatinous structures—rendering them more leather-like, and less susceptible to the corroding action of atmospheric oxygen, therefore less liable to waste or decay.

Most fruits contain, combined with the above-mentioned acids, *alkalies*, generally potash, which, on the combustion of the acids (citric, tartaric, etc.), are left in solution in the blood.

Alkalies increase the solubility of albumen and fibrin, and therefore tend to prevent undue fibrinous accumulation in or around the smaller bloodvessels.

Fruits contain very little nitrogen, as compared with the so-called nitrogenous or highly-nourishing foods. Many physiologists and physiological chemists have calculated the amount of nitrogen they think necessary to sustain life. This amount was dictated to them by experiments: these experiments were to find the amount *excreted* by the system.

It is a simple fact that the greater the quantity of nitrogen taken into the system, the greater is the amount eliminated; and it is very often observed in overfed people, that organs whose purpose is to eliminate nitrogenous products are unable to carry off any great excess, and free nitrogen is often eliminated by the skin.*

Therefore this process of inquiry cannot possibly give a correct result.

A proper estimate of the amount of nitrogen

* "It is further proved by the fact that the amount of nitrogen excreted is not in proportion to the work done, but to the quantity of it in the food, even when there is no muscular exertion."—LETHEBY.

DIET AND PROLONGED EXISTENCE. 97

required to sustain life can only be obtained by *direct* experiments—that is, living for a time on one class of food, then on another, and calculating the amount taken into the system, and the amount excreted, and during the time the experiments are carried on to weigh the body in order to ascertain loss or gain.[*] By this means a proximate amount required to keep the body in equilibrio may be obtained.

By experiments on ourselves, on friends, and on natives of tropical regions, including Western Africa, we find a comparatively small quantity of nitrogen necessary to sustain life in good bodily health—in fact, fruits, taken as a class, contain sufficient nitrogen to sustain human life.[†]

Many authors state that five or six ounces of gum[‡] (which contains carbon, hydrogen, oxygen, and little or no nitrogen), in the twenty-four hours, is sufficient to sustain life.

Adanson states that the nomadic Moors have scarcely any other food than gum-senegal, and Hasselquist asserts, that a caravan of Abyssinians, consisting of 1,000 persons, subsisted for two months on gum-arabic alone.

Humboldt relates that the natives on the coast of Caraccas prefer sugar[‡] to animal food, and we have

---

[*] The weight of the body is not necessarily a criterion of the value of food, because the weight may not alter, but water increase, and albumen and fat diminish in the system.

[†] The amount of nitrogen *excreted* is often greater than the amount *taken into* the system *as food and drink*.

[‡] *Impure* gum and *raw* sugar contain small quantities of nitrogen.

ourselves observed on the West Coast of Africa many tribes who subsist upon foods which contain comparatively little nitrogen.)

Plants absorb most of their *nitrogen* from the *air*. If a vegetable be supplied with ammonia (a compound of nitrogen and hydrogen), those parts of it which would, without it, be deposited as starch (which contains no nitrogen) become *gluten*, a substance which contains the same elements as albumen (carbon, hydrogen, oxygen, and nitrogen.

It has been urged that fruits will not sustain life because they do not contain sufficient nitrogen; this argument is founded upon a *theory* which is demonstrably incorrect, and it is an ascertained *fact* that fruits alone will support life in good bodily health.

The experiments of Macaire and Marcet prove that the blood contains more nitrogen than chyle.[*]

As the blood is formed from the chyle, the excess of nitrogen found in the blood must have another source than from the intestines, which source can only be the lungs or the skin, both of which are exposed to the atmosphere.

Sir Humphry Davy states, that in his experiments the absorption of nitrogen took place to the extent of 2,246 grains in the twenty-four hours.

When nitrogen comes in contact with hydrogen in a nascent state in an enclosed space, the two unite

---

[*] This can only be *partially* accounted for in the lacteals; after passing through the mesenteric glands, and receiving the lymph from the spleen, fat is decreased, fibrin increased, in their contents.

and form ammonia. Hydrogen is developed in the intestines and in the capillaries, therefore throughout the system wherever there is waste of tissue. It is possible that either ammonia, coming in contact with amylaceous substances destitute of nitrogen, or that these bodies, containing carbon, hydrogen, and oxygen, may unite directly with free nitrogen—the combination resulting in albumen or protein.

Now, fruits will sustain life, and all fruits contain carbon, hydrogen, and oxygen, and most of them a small quantity of nitrogen; and if these fruits which will sustain life do not contain sufficent nitrogen, may not man, who breathes and is in contact with an atmosphere four-fifths of which are nitrogen, by means of his lungs, the surface of which is supposed to be more than twenty times that of the whole body, absorb the necessary nitrogen directly from the atmosphere?

From careful observation on the diet of natives in tropical regions, and from direct experiments in England, we may state that this is positively the case.

This is often observed in the herbivora: their *natural* food contains little nitrogen, still it is found in their flesh to about the same extent as in the carnivora. Further, the carnivora live on food rich in nitrogen—yet one is as well nourished as the other.

Speaking of the *ancients*, Hesiod, the Greek poet says: "The uncultivated fields afforded them their *fruits*, and supplied their bountiful and unenvied repast."

Porphyry, a Platonic philosopher of the third century, a man of great talent and learning, says: "The ancient Greeks lived entirely upon the *fruits* of the earth."

Lucretius,* on the same subject, says:

> "Soft acorns were their first and chiefest food,
> And those red apples that adorn the wood.
> The nerves that joined their limbs were firm and strong;
> Their life was healthy, and their age was long. . . .
> Returning years still saw them in their prime;
> They wearied e'en the wings of measuring Time:
> Nor colds, nor heats, no strong diseases wait,
> And tell sad news of coming hasty fate:
> Nature not yet grew weak, not yet began
> To shrink into an inch the largest span."

Wherever we find animal life throughout Nature, we find its manifestation in development, growth, and nutrition depending upon the presence of albumen. The first visible state of an organised being is albumen; it is built up from albumen; its harder structures are caused by the oxidation of albumen; its food is albumen, which may (with the exception of what little may be formed† in the system) always be traced to, and was originally, vegetable albumen; if that food be vegetable food, this substance comes directly from the vegetable: if it be animal food, it comes originally from the vegetable through the medium of the animal.

"The continuance of life is indissolubly connected

---

* CREECH's translation.

† Formed in the system by the union of amylaceous substances with nitrogen.

DIET AND PROLONGED EXISTENCE.

with its presence in the blood—that is, in the nutrient fluid; only those substances are in a strict sense nutritious articles of food which contain either albumen, or a substance capable of being converted into albumen."—LIEBIG.

It *is* one of *Nature's laws*, and a very simple one, that we are built up from what originally was vegetable albumen; and with the exception of the alkaline and earthy salts, every structure and organ in our bodies was developed from and is nourished by albumen. It *was* one of the laws of Eden that man should eat albumen—vegetable albumen—in its purest form, as it exists in fruits.

There is, therefore, a simplicity, a reason, a wonderful philosophy in the first command given to man.

Man may live entirely upon fruits, in better health than the majority of mankind now enjoy. Good, sound, ripe fruits are never a cause of disease, but the vegetable acids, as we have before stated, *lower* the temperature of the body, decrease the process of combustion or oxidation—therefore the waste of the system—less sleep* is required, activity is increased, fatigue or thirst is hardly experienced: still the body is well nourished, and as a comparatively small quantity of earthy salts are taken into the system, the *cause* of "old age" is in some degree removed, the *effect* is delayed, and life is prolonged to a period far beyond our "threescore years and ten."

* "Adam's diet in the Garden was free from "old age producing matter." Chemically it was admirably adapted—not only to extraordinary longevity—but " to eat and live for ever." *(Original Eden.)*

HOW TO PROLONG LIFE.

Animal flesh, taken as a class, contains, next to fruits,* the least amount of earthy salts. The amount depends, *firstly*, upon the quantity contained in the food of the animal; *secondly*, upon the duration of time the animal has eaten such food—that is, its age. Younger animals of every class contain a less amount of earthy salts in their flesh than older ones; thus veal, in the analysis generally given, contains only about one-fourth the amount of earthy salts found in an equal weight of the flesh of an adult animal, and it further contains from 12 to 15 per cent. more phosphoric acid than is necessary for the formation of salts.

From this we see that the younger the animal, the less ossifying matter does its flesh contain; we should, therefore, select either growing animals or those just arrived at maturity, in preference to older animals, as a diet.

Amongst animal flesh we include *fish*. Those which have fins and scales contain, on an average, a per centage less salts (about ·7) than animal flesh, and are, therefore, to a certain extent, better adapted as a diet to longevity than butcher's meat. Fish also contains phosphorus; this is especially marked in most shell-fish, which, however, contain more earthy matter than fish with fins and scales.

* On one occasion, when living for five days entirely upon *oranges*, our temperature was lessened, still we felt a pleasant glow throughout the system; but to other individuals we felt cold. Animal heat is therefore only *relative*; we found further that only three or four hours' sleep was required in the twenty-hours.

The flesh of poultry and game (if young) contains less earthy salts than beef or mutton.

Animal flesh without fat will support life; gelatine or jelly, although containing nearly as much nitrogen as muscular fibre, will not: the reason is that digestion is incapable of converting it into albumen. Dogs fed on gelatine also soon died, but they have lived many months on pure albuminous matter.

"The true unsophisticated American Indians near the sources of the Missouri, during the winter months, are reported to subsist entirely upon dried buffalo flesh—not the fat portions, but the muscular part. . . . During their subsistence on dried *pemmican*, they are described by travellers, who are intimate with their habits of life, as never tasting even the most minute portions of any vegetable whatever, or partaking of any other variety of food. These facts, then, tend to show that *albuminous* tissue is of *itself* capable of sustaining life."—DR. THOMPSON.

In other articles of animal food we have *milk*, unskimmed, skimmed, and butter-milk; they all contain about ·7 per cent. of salts; but the latter contains a large quantity of lactic acid, which has a great tendency to prevent the accumulation of earthy matter in the system.

Cheese contains salt in about the same proportion as milk deprived of its water. It seems by its analysis to have a large quantity of salts (nearly 5 per cent.), but they exist in ratio to its highly nourishing properties.

HOW TO PROLONG LIFE.

Butter is composed of fat, and contains about 2 per cent. of salts. It is not a fat either formed or altered in the animal economy. It may be artificially produced from grass, and may therefore be termed the "fat of the land."

Eggs contain 1·5 per cent. of salts (·5 per cent. less than beef and mutton).

We will now briefly consider the *vegetable roots*. The potato contains 9 per cent. of salts, 1·4 of albuminous matter, and 15·5 of starch; it contains sugar, a small quantity of fat, and a small proportion of free citric acid.

The onion is very nutritious, and it contains small quantities of phosphate of lime, but there is an *excess* of phosphoric acid; also mucilage, and a substance analagous to gluten.

Most other *roots* contain a large quantity of water, and, in proportion to their nutrient properties, a large quantity of fibrous and earthy matter. Most other *vegetables* have about the same nourishing properties as the potato, about the same amount of earthy salts,* but contain more water and less starch. The cucumber and fungi are exceptions, and are similar to fruit.

* The amount of earthy salts they contain depends entirely upon the soil in which they are grown. If we take one dram of cress-seed, incinerate it, and weigh the amount of salt it contains; and if we take another dram of the same seed, and place it on flannel (which has been soaked for some weeks in distilled water to free it from soluble salts) in a vessel, and fill the vessel with distilled water to a level with the flannel, the seeds will grow and become plants, almost as perfect as if grown in soil; if we then dry and incinerate these plants, they are

We now come to the *cereals*, in which we will include the leguminous seeds. The amount of earthy matter they contain depends upon the amount contained in the soil, or in substances used as manure.

The cereals constitute the basis of man's food; they mostly contain large quantities of mineral matter, and as a class are the worst adapted as a food for man, in regard to a long life. Man's so-called "staff of life" is, to a great extent, the cause of his premature death.

"The system obtains its supply of *earthy* substances from both animal and vegetable foods. *Corn, potatoes, milk,* and the *flesh* and *blood* of animals *furnish* us with *more than the wants of the system require*."—DR. PEREIRA.

In the twenty-second and twenty-third chapters of the third book ("Thalia") of Herodotus, describing a visit of some Persian Ambassadors to the long-lived Ethiopians (Macrobii*), the Ethiopians "asked what the Persian King was wont to eat, and to what age

---

found to contain exactly the same amount of salts as that existing in the seed from which they grew. The salts previously contained in the seeds have been, by the process of growth, distributed in the substance of the plants. Starchy goods do not, as generally stated, contain the largest percentage of lime.

* "Macrobii, a people of Æthiopia, celebrated for their justice and the innocence of their manners. They generally lived to their one hundred and twentieth year, some say to a thousand; and, indeed, from that longevity they have obtained their name ($\mu\alpha\kappa\rho o s$ $\beta\iota o s$, *long life*) to distinguish them more particularly from the other inhabitants of Æthiopia. After so long a period spent in virtuous actions, and freed from the indulgence of vice, and from maladies, they dropped into the grave as to sleep, without pain or terror."—LEMPRIERE.

the longest-lived of the Persians had been known to attain. They told him that the King ate *bread*, and described the nature of *wheat*—adding that *eighty years* was the longest term of man's life among the Persians. Hereat he remarked, 'It did not surprise him, if they fed on *dirt* (bread), that they died so soon; indeed, he was sure they never would have lived so long as eighty years except for the refreshment they got from that drink (meaning the wine), wherein he confessed the Persians surpassed the Ethiopians.' The Ichthyophagi then, in their turn, questioned the King concerning the term of life and diet of his people, and were told that most of them lived to be *a hundred and twenty years old*, while some even went beyond that age: they ate *boiled flesh*, and had for their drink nothing but *milk*."

"Notwithstanding that bread is denominated the *staff of life*, alone it does *not* appear to be *capable* of supporting *prolonged human existence*. Boussingault came to this conclusion from observing the small quantity of nitrogen which it contains; and the Reports of the Inspectors of Prisons, on the effect of a diet of bread and water, favour this opinion."— PEREIRA.

Majendie fed a dog exclusively on fine wheaten bread—it died in forty days; whilst another dog, fed on black bread (brown bread—flour with the bran), lived without any disturbance in good health.

The nutrient part of wheat is chiefly gluten. *Bran* is rich in gluten, and should therefore *not be removed*.

Whole-meal bread, however, contains more phosphate of lime than white.

Leguminous seeds (peas, beans, etc.) are supposed to be less nutritive than the cereals, although the former contain more nitrogen than the latter. This Liebig attributes to a deficiency of *earthy phosphates*, which, however, could not be the reason, as Broconnot gives *peas* as containing 9·26 grains per ounce of earthy phosphates. This is nearly twice the quantity found in wheat, and more than twenty times the amount in an equal weight of beef.

Phosphoric acid and the alkalies have both of them remarkable properties, and play an important part in the growth and nutrition of plants and animals.

This cannot be said of the *earthy* salts. They develop the bones of animals, but when this is accomplished they accumulate and cause the ossification of "old age"—even "natural death."

We should, therefore, after we arrive at muturity, avoid as much as possible *earthy* salts in our food.

Many interesting and well-conducted experiments of agricultural chemists agree, and give the following facts:

1. Vegetables and cereals grown in soil containing a small percentage of *earthy* salts, contain a less amount than those grown in soil rich in earthy salts.

2. The greater the quantity of earthy salts contained in the food on which an animal subsists, the greater is the amount found in the secretions and

excretions, and the greater is the amount found in the *flesh* of the animal.

3. The less the amount of earthy salts in the food, the less the amount found in the secretions and excretions, and the less the amount in the flesh. The result of these experiments thus favours in the abstract what we adopt in the principle.

From these facts it is clear, that in growing cereals and vegetables directly for the consumption of man, or indirectly for the food of animals on which he partly subsists, *Lime or any of its compounds should not be used as a manure.* Alkalies do not accumulate in the system; there is, therefore, no objection to their use.

We, therefore, see that the different kinds of food, in regard to longevity, have the following order : *fruits, fish, animal food* (flesh, eggs, etc.), *vegetables, cereals.*

In the same order do we trace the age of man by his diet. It is written that man in the first ages lived for a period which to us seems incredible; but in the present generation the average time of life is so short, that a man at eighty or ninety years is truly a modern " patriarch." Man's first and ordained diet was fruits; he then eat animal food, which was subsequently permitted to him; after this he gained a knowledge of agriculture—he grew vegetables and cereals; and not content with this, during the last few years he has learned to add lime artificially to them—to shrink and lessen an already shortened existence.

DIET AND PROLONGED EXISTENCE.

In Nature a curious yet simple phenomenon is often observed—a *rise* and *fall*. If perpetual, it alternates and becomes a fall and rise. We notice it in the sun, in gravity, in fluctuation, in the tides. and even in the rise and fall of empires.

Man has degenerated—this degeneration is due solely to his diet. He has *fallen*; but we hope that he has *risen* to the highest point in the art of shortening his days, and that in the present generation he will commence to gradually *fall* back on his original and ordained diet. Since the creation, the days of man's existence have been little by little decreasing—it has been a gradual *fall*; but both science and religion tell us that he must *rise* again, that his life on earth must be prolonged. *This can only be accomplished by a gradual alteration in his diet.*

Let us imagine a man, who is a great smoker, suddenly deprived of tobacco. What would be his feelings?

Let us picture to ourselves a man, enjoying all the luxuries and enjoyments of modern life, suddenly deprived of them. What would be his feelings? They would both be for a time wretched and miserable.

It is not our purpose to dictate a course which would have a similar result. Our purpose is, by pointing out a method of gradually altering diet, to endeavour to improve and benefit humanity, and to lengthen the days and increase the happiness of man.

"Nature is frugal, and her wants are few." Man in the savage state is generally healthy, in the *civilized* state he is generally unhealthy: and, as Dr. Thompson says, "There is no doubt that a simple diet is more fitted to accelerate health than unnatural and stimulating foods." It is not necessary that man should return to the savage state in order that he should enjoy health, nor does it follow that because man in his wild state is healthy, civilized man should be diseased; particularly when he awakens to the fact that diet is the great cause of his sufferings, and that the antidote rests to a great extent with himself—that the nearer he approaches to his original diet, the more healthy will he be.

"We cannot expect a nation to bound and stride into perfection at once. It is only by slow painful efforts that a nation works out its redemption from darkness and ignorance."—LORD ROSEBERY.

It would be a difficult task, and a great tax on the system, for a man who lives on an ordinary mixed diet to suddenly change it. He must do this gradually; and in direct ratio as he does this will the tendency to disease decrease, and the prospect of long life increase.

If we look at the ordinary articles of diet, we notice to a great extent the following principle: that the more nitrogenous substances—*direct* nourishment —a food contains, the more earthy salts are there found in it; and the less the nourishment, the less the amount of earthy salts in the food.

It is a well-known fact that the more nitrogenous substances a food contains, the less is the amount required to nourish the body; and inversely, the less the amount of these substances, the greater is the amount required to sustain life. If we take cheese and rice as an example, the former contains far more nitrogen, also far more earthy salts than the latter. But a small quantity of cheese will support life, whilst in order to live on rice, a man must eat a large quantity; so that one man whilst eating a small quantity of cheese, rich in nitrogen and earthy salts, another, living on rice, must eat a proportionately large quantity; and in the end both consume about the same amount of nitrogenous substances, and about the same amount of earthy salts. Fruits are the great exception to this rule, but others are observed: as, for instance, one man subsists on bread, another, we will say, on mutton. In order to obtain the same nourishment in both cases, the bread-eater would have to eat more than twice the quantity consumed by the other, and he would further take into his system two and a half times more earthy salts than the flesh-eater. Lentils are another exception; and in proportion to their nourishing properties, they contain only one-third the amount of earthy salts as compared with bread.

Before selecting a diet, or giving any rules thereon, a word on the question of quantity is requisite. One authority says "that a full-grown man of average weight (140 to 150 lbs.), and height (5 ft.

7 in.), requires *one-twentieth* part of his weight in food during the twenty-four hours; that is, *seven or seven and a half pounds* of food, including solids and liquids, *one to one and a half pound* (sixteen to twenty-four ounces) being *solids*, the rest water."

Another authority says *eight pounds of food* are required daily, *two pounds* of which must be *solid*, the remaining *six pounds liquid*.

Now these results are arrived at by *indirect* experiment, determining the waste; and we have before pointed out that this principle of inquiry cannot possibly give a correct result, because the greater the amount of food and drink a man takes into his system, the greater will be the amount of solids, liquids, and gases excreted and eliminated by the body. *Direct* experiment only will give us a correct result, and we have positive evidence to show that little more than half the above quantities of solids are necessary to keep the body *in equilibrio*—to sustain life.

"It may with truth be asserted that the greater part of mankind eat more than is necessary; and by being crammed and over-fed in infancy, we are deprived of that natural sensation which ought to tell us when we have enough."—HUFELAND.

A good instance of this is seen in the well-known case of Louis Cornaro, who, "till the fortieth year of his age, had led a life of dissipation . . . and was so far reduced that his physician assured him he could not live above two months; that all medicines would

DIET AND PROLONGED EXISTENCE. 113

be useless, and that the only thing which could be recommended for him was a *spare diet*. Having followed this advice, he found, after some days, he was much better; and at the end of a few years his health was not only perfectly re-established, but he became sounder than ever he had been before . . . For *sixty whole years* he took no more than *twelve ounces of food*, everything included, and *thirteen ounces of drink*, daily . . . When he was eighty years of age, his friends prevailed upon him to make a little addition to his food . . . ; he gave way to their request, and raised his food to fourteen, and his drink to sixteen ounces. 'Scarcely,' says he, 'had I continued this mode of living ten days, when I began, instead of being cheerful and lively as before, to become uneasy and dejected, a burden to myself and to others. . . . But by the blessing of God, and my *former regimen*, I recovered; and now, in my eighty-third year, I enjoy a happy state of body and mind. I can climb steep hills . . . and I am a stranger to those peevish and morose humours which fall so often to the lot of old age.'· In this happy disposition he attained his hundredth year."— HUFELAND.

"A cheerful and a good heart will have a care for his meat and diet." Gluttony is truly a sin, not legally punishable, but revengeful in itself on the individual; it is the cause of a distinct debility from loss of nerve-power in digesting excess of food, and the sufferer, although gormandising and eating ravenously, becomes thinner and thinner, weaker and weaker, and in his efforts to nourish his pining frame, he creeps nearer and nearer to the jaws of *premature death.*

Obesity is sometimes caused by over-eating, but this is not always the case, for we see many corpulent persons who are very small eaters. Want of proper exercise is the commoner cause.

Many diseases have excessive eating solely as a cause. Remove the cause, the effect cannot follow. A state of bodily equilibrium, which we will designate by the word *health*, is the result of a conformity to the laws of Nature; apart from this, there can only be the conditions *plus* and *minus*—excess or deficiency; and where either of these diverges to any considerable extent, we have *disease.*

Although thoroughly acquainted with the effects of deficient food, on inquiry we are bound to come to the conclusion that many cases of starvation—the results of famine or insufficient nourishment—are often due to the *quality*, more than the *quantity*, of food.

Dr. Aitken quotes the following diet of a labourer under the old "truck system," which was often the cause of outbreaks of *scurvy*: "His daily diet consisted of *one pennyworth of bread, with tea, but no milk, in the morning; no dinner; and one pennyworth of bread, with tea, and no milk, in the evening.* After existing *three months* on this diet, the disease broke out." What else could be expected? Bread *alone* is not a proper diet for man. Had he added to it but

DIET AND PROLONGED EXISTENCE.

a small quantity of his original, ordained, and best adapted diet—fruits, experience tells us he would not have been afflicted.

White bread and gelatine are popularly supposed to be very nutritious. Now a man may feed an animal on bread and gelatine, and under the erroneous impression that he is feeding the animal well, give it pounds a day, but many experiments tell us that in time the animal will die of starvation —deficiency of *proper* nourishing food.

Did man know the *quality* of foods, had he the power of discriminating why he should eat this and avoid that, he would be able to live on far less than he at present does, and he would further be less subject to disease. For this reason we think that it is requisite that every child should be taught at school, and should be made acquainted with, the elements of himself and the food by which his body is nourished, in the full impression that his well-being depends more upon this knowledge than a study of the dead languages and theoretical sciences.

This reminds us that as yet we have not mentioned childhood, but as our remarks are chiefly confined to those arrived at maturity, a lengthy discourse on the subject is unnecessary. A few words, however, may not be out of place. In the word "childhood" we will include that period of life which commences in infancy (at birth), and extends to early adult age (maturity). We therefore speak of that time of life during which the development of the different organs and textures is proceeding, and their functions becoming more perfect; during which, also, the mental manifestations, intellectual, moral, and emotional, develop and gain strength. In infancy, or commencing childhood, the functions are chiefly vegetative, and the movements, to a great extent, automatic, and during this period all the organs, particularly the osseous, nervous, and locomotory systems, are in a state of development. During this period the infant's food is *milk*.

In infancy, nourishment is required for the growth of the soft structures—*albumen* will answer this purpose; also for the hard structures, cartilage and bone —*chondrine* and the salts contained in milk will do all that is necessary.

The nutrient part of milk is chiefly its *caseine*, and if to the formula of caseine be added ten eqs. of oxygen, we obtain a formula which contains exactly the same elements as the albumen of blood and chondrine.

The formulæ as given by Liebig are:

	Sulphur. Eqs.	Nitrogen. Eqs.	Carbon. Eqs.	Hydrogen. Eqs.	Oxygen. Eqs.
The formula of *chondrine* is .	—	9	72	59	32
Add the formula of *albumen* of blood.	2	27	216	169	68
Total .	2	36	288	228	100
Together = the formula of *caseine* (of milk)	2	36	288	228	90
+ 10 eqs. of oxygen.	—	—	—	—	10

DIET AND PROLONGED EXISTENCE. 117

The oxygen the child readily gets from the atmosphere by the process of respiration, and if to this we add the salts, alkaline and earthy, contained in milk, we find albumen as the chief constituent of its blood —the developing and nutrient fluid of every organ and structure; chondrine and salts, to develop its cartilages and bones. Thus in milk Nature supplies childhood with all its wants, and for this reason milk is a food better fitted to childhood than adult life.

It is a well-known fact that children brought up on *human* milk are healthier and more robust than children fed on cow's milk. The reason is obvious. The salts in *human milk* exist in ratio to its nourishing properties, as one part of salts to seventeen and a half parts of nitrogenous matter; in *cow's* milk, as one part of salts to six and one-third parts of the same nourishing substances. Therefore, in round numbers, the nutrient part of cow's milk contains nearly three times the amount of salts as compared with human milk. The proportions of alkaline and earthy salts are proximately the same in the ashes of both, so that one ounce of caseine taken from cow's milk contains nearly three times the amount of *earthy* salts found in an equal weight of caseine from human milk.

A human being takes four or five times longer to mature than a cow; the latter therefore grows more quickly, and its bones ossify in a less period of time than the former, whose organs are more gradual in their development and growth—whose bones should take a longer time to ossify, and therefore Nature gives a food which contains less *earthy* matter. If we do not follow Nature's laws, some bad result must follow, and one-half of our strumous children, who, besides their milk, are, as a rule, fed on bread and other farinaceous foods—most of them rich in earthy compounds—are for their age, in years and months, bodily older than healthy and robust children of the same age.

Rickets and mollities ossium are in themselves diseases, not necessarily caused by a deficiency of earthy salts in the food, but by a lack in the system of power to assimilate them, or to their solution by acid.

We can stunt the growth of the lower animals by giving them an excess of earthy matter; we can ossify them, make them permanently old, and shorten their days, by the same. In human beings we need not look further than the Cretins found in the valleys of the Alps, Pyrenees, and other regions. Although cretinism has two* distinct causes, the first and most important is that an excess of *earthy* matter—lime or *magnesian lime*—is taken into the system in solution in water used for drinking purposes. Hereditary it

* The other cause is an electro-magnetic action, due to the peculiar *geological* formations in some districts where cretinism prevails, and which influences the excretion of earthy salts from the system. For there are many recorded cases of this disease where the afflicted persons did not use lime or *hard* water—in fact, where the water was *soft*, the sufferers eating the same or a similar diet to persons free from the disease but not resident in the district. Both, therefore, take into their systems about the same amount of calcareous salts, but the one *excretes* nearly the whole, the other *retains* the same.

DIET AND PROLONGED EXISTENCE. 119

must be to children born of parents suffering from this disease, if not removed from the cause; but sound healthy children brought into districts where cretinism exists, are, at an early age, equally subject to the disease with children born in them.

Now these beings are, in their infancy, literally prematurely ossified; the development of the bones is arrested, the height being seldom more than four and a half feet. The bones of the cranium, which in a natural state should expand to allow the brain to grow and develop, at an early age become thickened, hardened, and ossified to such an extent that expansion is impossible; the brain, therefore, cannot develop; it is gradually deprived of its blood-supply from below; it is encased and imprisoned by its own shield; its intellectual part cannot develop; the being is subservient to the animal portion; he becomes voracious and lascivious, and in many cases sinks in intelligence below the level of many of the brutes. The age of Cretins is short; few of them reach thirty years, and, as Clayton remarks, " although they die early, they soon present the appearance of age." This miserable state of existence is due, to a great extent, to *premature* ossification.

It is therefore clear that infants should be fed on *human* milk; that children, during their growth, should not be fed almost entirely on foods rich in earthy salts—on a cereal or farinaceous diet; time should be given for the expansion and development of their bodies. They should, therefore, eat a mixed diet—fruits or animal food in excess of the farinaceous; and further, as use determines the shape of a limb, exercise and athletic games should be encouraged; and as the *mind* influences the character, sympathies, and welfare of man, and places him by its activity and development at the head of all animated creation, education—the fountain of intellectual manifestations, of sound principles of action and conduct, of the elegancies, accomplishments, and endearments of life—should be carried out in a manner which will be attractive to, and appreciated by, the receiver of *knowledge*; so that in decomposing the information thus acquired, and recombining it in useful and attractive forms, he may lay the foundation in learning, from the supervision and experience of the good, and upon it construct a castle of *wisdom*—but not at the expense of bodily health.

> "*Knowledge* and *Wisdom*, far from being one,
> Have ofttimes no connection. *Knowledge* dwells
> In heads replete with thoughts of other men;
> *Wisdom* in minds attentive to their own.
> *Knowledge*, a rude unprofitable mass,
> The mere materials with which *Wisdom* builds,
> Till smooth'd, and squar'd, and fitted to its place,
> Doth but encumber whom it seems t' enrich.
> *Knowledge* is proud that he has learn'd so much;
> *Wisdom* is humble that she knows no more."
>
> COWPER.

To return to the subject of *quantity* of food required to sustain life, we affirm that most men eat **more than** is requisite for this purpose—more than is

DIET AND PROLONGED EXISTENCE.

actually good for them. Man does not require four or five meals a day; he would be in far better health on two, or at most three, meals in the twenty-four hours.

Fruits are nutritious in themselves; but should they not contain sufficient nitrogen to satisfy a *theoretical* appetite, we have shown that all other elements are present, and that man may absorb the deficient nitrogen from the surrounding atmosphere, the combination resulting in albumen, or protein. For this reason, together with the fact that they contain little earthy matter, fruits are man's best diet if he truly desires a long life; but considering the difficulties attending a sudden change of diet, and the necessity of conforming to the rules and usages of society, which we do not wish to usurp (and even did we desire this, we fear society would be the victor), we are induced to put forward a few *simple* and straightforward *rules*, which are founded upon observed facts, which are not oppressive or tyrannical, which would not interfere with the avocations and callings of man, and which may be readily carried out by every one of the community for his own individual benefit, for health and long life.

As we know there are many who could not be persuaded to make any alteration in the *articles* of their diet, whilst there are others who might be influenced in this direction, we give a few rules for both these classes.

To those who are not inclined to alter the articles of their diet, we say:

1. Eat *moderately*, always remembering that you eat to live—to give a balance to the system.
2. Take no more than three meals a day.
3. *Avoid* eating *large quantities* of bread, pastry, and other farinaceous foods.

To those who are willing to make alterations in their diet, the same rules will apply, but with this difference:

Eat *fruits*, if possible, at every meal, and commence with them; if the appetite is not moderately satisfied, finish with the ordinary articles of diet.

A fruit diet gives to a great extent freedom from disease.

CHAPTER IV.

INSTANCES OF LONGEVITY IN MAN AND IN THE ANIMAL AND VEGETABLE KINGDOMS.

ON reviewing nearly two thousand reported cases of persons who lived more than a century, we generally find some peculiarity of diet or habits to account for their alleged longevity; we find some were living amongst all the luxuries life could afford, others in the most abject poverty—begging their bread; some were samples of symmetry and physique, others cripples; some drank large quantities of water, others little; some were total abstainers from alcoholic drinks, others drunkards; some smoked tobacco, others did not; some lived entirely on vegetables, others to a great extent on animal foods; some led active lives, others sedentary; some worked with their brain, others with their hands; some ate only one meal a day, others four or five; some few ate large quantities of food, others a small amount; in fact, we notice great divergence both in habits and diet, but in those cases where we have been able to obtain a reliable account of the diet, we find one *great cause* which accounts for the majority of cases of longevity, *moderation in the quantity of food.*

To illustrate this, we append a few cases from Easton, Hufeland, Bailey, and other authors. Some may be exaggerated, and to be received *cum grano salis*. We give them to illustrate a principle:

Judith Bannister, of Cowes, Isle of Wight, died in 1754, aged 108.

"She lived upon biscuit and *apples*, with milk and water, the last sixty years of her life."

Ann Maynard, of Finchley, died in 1756, aged 112.

"She lived with *moderation*, and took much exercise."

John Michaelstone (grandson of Thomas Parr), died in 1763, aged 127.

"He lived to the above great age by *extreme temperance.*"

Owen Carollan, of Duleck, county Meath, died in 1764, aged 127.

"By *temperance* and hard labour he attained so great an age."

Janet Anderson, of Newington, Middlesex, died in 1764, aged 102.

"Her life was *regular and moderate.*"

Elizabeth Macpherson, lived in the county of Caithness, died in 1765, aged 117.

"Her diet was *buttermilk and greens;* she retained all her senses till within three months of her death."

Mr. Dobson, of Hatfield, farmer, died in 1766, aged 139.

"By much exercise and *temperate living* he preserved the inestimable blessing of health."

Francis Confit, of Burythorpe, near Malton, Yorkshire, died in 1767, aged 150.

"He was *very temperate in his living*, and used great exercise, which, together with occasionally eating a *raw* egg, enabled him to attain such extraordinary age."

Catherine Noon *alias* Noony, lived near the city of Tuam, in Ireland, died the same year, aged 136.

"Was *very temperate at her meals*. Her husband died aged 128."

Philip Loutier, of Shoreditch, London, a French barber, died at 105.

"He drank nothing but water, and *ate only once a day*."

Donald M'Gregor, a farmer in the Isle of Skye, died at 117.

"*He was temperate at his meals*, and took much exercise."

Mrs. Boyce, of Guildford, Surrey, died in 1771, aged 107.

"By *temperance* she acquired constant health."

Paul Barral, of Nice, a priest, died in 1771, aged 106.

"He continued in good health by living on vegetables."

Mrs. Keithe, of Newnham, Gloucestershire, died in 1772, aged 133.

"She *lived moderately*, and retained her senses till within fourteen days of her death.

Mrs. Clum, lived near Lichfield, Staffordshire, died in 1773, aged 138.

"By frequent exercise and *temperate living* she attained so great longevity . . . she resided in the same house 103 years."

Mary Rogers, of Penzance, Cornwall, died in 1779, aged 118.

"Lived the last sixty years on *vegetables*."

Fluellyn Price, of Glamorgan, died the same year, aged 101.

"Possessed a great flow of spirits, attended with sound health and activity, which blessings were the result of his *abstemious manner of living*. Herb teas were his breakfast, meat plainly dressed his dinner, and *instead* of a supper, he refreshed himself with smoking a pipe of tobacco."

Joseph Ekins, of Coombe, Berks, labourer, died in 1780, aged 103.

"Never suffered a week's illness, and for the last forty years subsisted entirely on bread, milk, and *vegetables*."

Henry Grosvenor, of Inch, county Wexford, a gentleman of French extraction, surveyor of the coast of Blackwater, died in 1780, aged 115.

"*He was very sparing in his diet*, and used much exercise, and was an agreeable, cheerful companion at one hundred, when he married his last wife."

Val. Coleby, of Preston, near Hull, died in 1782, aged 116.

"His diet for twenty years was milk and biscuit."

Edward Drinker, of Philadelphia, died in 1782, aged 103.

INSTANCES OF LONGEVITY.

"He lived on very solid food, drank tea in the afternoon, but *ate no supper.*"

Alexander Mackintosh, of Marseilles, died at 112.

"For the last ten years he lived *entirely on vegetables*, and enjoyed a good state of health till within two days of his death."

James Le Measurer, of St. Jean Pied de Port, in Navarre, died in 1784, aged 118.

"His common food for some years was *vegetables.*"

Lewis Morgan, of Llwringtdod, Radnorshire, died at 101.

"His death was occasioned by a fall . . . he lived chiefly on *vegetable diet.*"

Mr. Smith, of Dolver, Montgomeryshire, farmer, died in 1785, aged 103.

"He was never known to drink anything but *buttermilk.*"

Cardinal de Salis, Archbishop of Seville, died the same year, aged 125.

He himself observed : "I led a sober, studious, but not a lazy or sedentary life. My *diet was sparing*, though delicate ; my liquors the best wines of Xeres and La Mancha, of which I never exceeded a pint at any meal, except in cold weather, when I allowed myself one-third more."

Margaret M'Carthy, of Cork, died in 1789, aged 103.

"She lived *abstemiously*, and was very regular at her *meals.*"

Anne Bannerman died the same year at Aberdeen, aged 105.

"She latterly subsisted on *vegetables* and small beverage."

John Ursulak, a silk weaver, of Limburg, Prussia, died in 1812, aged 116.

" He was of *temperate* and sober habits."

John Wilson, of Worlingworth, Sussex, died in 1782, aged 116.

" For the last forty years of his life his suppers were almost uniformly made out of roasted *turnips* ; to which vegetable, thus prepared, he always ascribed peculiar sanitary virtues."

Bernard le Borier de Fontanelle, of Rouen, France, died in 1757, aged 100. He was a man of great talent, was Dean of the French Academy, Fellow of the Royal Society of London and of the Royal Academy of Berlin.

"Till upwards of ninety he does not appear to have experienced any of the maladies usually attendant upon old age. After this time he was subject to a periodical attack of fever in the spring, when he used to say, ' If I can only hold out till *strawberries* come in I shall get well.' He always *attributed his longevity* to a good *course of strawberry eating* every season."

Petratsch Zartan died in 1724, aged 185 years. He was born in 1537, at Kofroek, a village three miles from Temeswaer, in Hungary, where he lived 180 years.

"Being a member of the Greek Church, the old man was a strict observer of the numerous *fasts* established by its ritual, and was at all times *very abstemious in his diet*, save that once a day, with the milk and leaven cakes which constituted his sole food, he took a good-sized glass of brandy."

Galen, a physician of Pergamus, died about A.D. 270, aged 140.

He himself informs us that he always *ate* and drank *sparingly*, irrespective of his appetite, and although of delicate constitution, he attributed his longevity to his temperance.

Henry Hastings, Esq., second son of the Earl of Huntingdon, died in 1650, aged 109.

He was an original character, a great sportsman, and "never failed to eat *oysters* both at dinner and supper."

Marie Mallet, of Thènezay, France, died in 1845, aged 115.

"She was always very *abstemious* in her habits."

William Mead, M.D. (possibly grandfather of the celebrated Dr. Mead), died at Ware, Herts, in 1652, aged 148.

"He was distinguished for his great *temperance* and regular habits of life."

Mary Meigan, of Donaghmore, Ireland, died in 1813, aged 129.

"During the last thirty years of her life she lived apparently in the greatest penury and distress, *scarcely affording herself the means necessary for the keeping together of soul and body*." She, however, saved £1,600.

Mr. R. Bowman, of Irthdington, near Carlisle, died in 1823, aged 118.

Bailey says: "He never used tea or coffee; his principal diet was bread, potatoes, hasty pudding, broth, and occasionally a little flesh meat. He scarcely ever tasted ale or spirits; his principal beverage was water, or milk and water mixed. It is, however, right, to state that this *extreme abstemiousness*, in all probability, arose as much from the desire to accumulate money as from the love of temperance."

Mrs. Barnett, widow, of Edgeworth Town, Ireland, died in 1809, aged 116.

"In her habits of *diet* she was always *very temperate*."

Bridget Devine, of Alean Street, Manchester, died in 1845, aged 147.

Her husband was a handloom weaver, and died about twenty years before her. They were *very poor*, and after her husband's decease she was *supported* chiefly from the *parochial funds*.

Ephraim Pratt was living at Shaftesbury, U.S., in 1803, aged 116.

The Rev. T. Dwight states that this man was born at Sudbury, Mass., in 1687, and that throughout his life he had been *very temperate*, both in *diet* and habits. His general drink was *cider*; he was accustomed to take animal food, but in *less quantity* than most persons around him. Milk was also a common article of his diet.

INSTANCES OF LONGEVITY.

The Hon. Mrs. Watkins, of Glamorganshire, died in 1790, aged 110.

"She was remarkable for regularity and *moderation*. For the last thirty years she subsisted entirely on potatoes."

Jonathan Hartop, of the village of Aldborough, near Boroughbridge, Yorkshire, died in 1790, aged 138.

"*He ate but little*, and his only beverage was milk."

Rebecca Joseph, of Malpas, near Newport, Monmouth, died the same year, aged 100.

"She lived a very *temperate life*. Her chief sustenance for the last two years was brown sugar and cold water."

Anne Froste, of West Raisin, Lincolnshire, died in 1722, aged 111.

"Married her last husband in her ninety-third year. . . . For many years past she had lived on *milk and tea diet*."

Mr. Sherwood, of Stokesley, in Cleveland, died in 1794, aged 105.

"By using much exercise, and by *temperate living*, he enjoyed an unusual share of good health."

Mrs. Thomson, lived near Dublin, died in 1796, aged 135.

"She was very active; and by a *regular mode of living*, together with much exercise, attained so great age."

A labourer, named Stender, died in 1792, in the Duchy of Holstein, aged 103.

"His food, for the most part, was nothing but oatmeal and *buttermilk*."

Baron Baravicio de Capellis, died in 1770, at Meran, in Tyrol, aged 104.

"His usual food was *eggs*; he never tasted boiled flesh; sometimes he ate a little roasted, but always in *very small quantity*; and he drank abundance of tea with rosa-solis, and sugar-candy."

Charles Macklin, of James Street, Covent Garden, an eminent dramatic writer, and comedian of Covent Garden Theatre, the veteran father of the stage, died in 1797, aged 107. In the former part of his life he lived intemperately; subsequent thereto, he determined to proceed by rule, which he scrupulously observed.

"*He was moderate at his meals*, and ate fish, flesh, etc., till the age of seventy; when finding tea did not agree with him, he substituted milk, with a little bread boiled in it, sweetened with brown sugar. . . . For the last forty years, his principal beverage was white wine and water, pretty sweet. . . . He strictly observed the dictates of nature, ate when hungry, drank when thirsty, and slept when sleepy."—*Vide* Memoirs of his life.

"DEATH OF A CENTENARIAN DOCTOR.—Dr. Severin Wielobycki, a Polish refugee, who was born on January 8, 1793, and had for many years resided in England, died on Thursday, at his residence, Acacia Road, St. John's Wood, of embolism, following a third attack of influenza. The son of a judge in Poland, Severin Wielobycki fought as a captain in a volunteer cavalry regiment, in the last struggle for Poland, in 1830, and was engaged in thirty-six battles. On the collapse of the rising he had to fly the country, and his father was for a time imprisoned on suspicion of being privy to his escape. Taking refuge in Edinburgh, he applied himself to the study of English and medicine, at the same time supporting himself by teaching French. It was not until he had resided in Edinburgh for ten years, that he was able to enter the University, and he was 52 when he graduated M.D. there, in 1841. He subsequently went to Nova Scotia, where he practised medicine for some time, also in Leicester and Camberwell. Retiring twenty-seven years ago, he settled in St. John's Wood, and till two years ago was in the habit of walking twelve miles every day, and being at the top of Primrose Hill every morning at five o'clock, both in winter and summer. Vegetarians, anti-tobacconists, and teetotallers will no doubt ascribe his longevity to the facts that he had never used tobacco, that he had not tasted alcohol for forty years, and that for seventeen years he had been a vegetarian. At least, he himself attributed his length of days to these circumstances, in the course of a speech which he made at a reception given in honour of his centenary by the Society for the Study of Inebriety, in January last. Except that latterly he was very deaf, deceased sustained all his faculties to the last, and was able to read small type without the aid of glasses. He contributed to some of the medical papers, and was a member of the British Medical Temperance Association, in the work of which he took much interest."—*The People*, 1893.

In the following cases, moderation and temperance may have been practised in diet, but not in alcoholic drinks and tobacco :

Daniel Bull McCarthy, lived in the county of Kerry, Ireland, died in 1752, aged 111.

"For the last seventy years, when in company, he drank *plentifully* of *rum* and *brandy*, which he called *naked truth*, and if, in compliance with solicitations, he drank claret or punch, he always drank an equal glass of rum or brandy, which he called a *wedge*."

Thomas Whittington, of Heillingdon, Middlesex, died in 1804, aged 104.

"Actually never took any other liquids, as liquids, into his stomach than ardent spirit—London gin ; of which compound, until within a fortnight of his death, he took from a pint to a pint and a half daily."

"George Kirton, Esq., of Oxnop Hall, Yorkshire, died in 1764, aged 125.

He was a great foxhunter, and "no man, till within ten years of his death, made more free with the bottle."

Philip Laroque, of Frie, in Gascony, butcher, died in 1766, aged 102.

"Was drunk regularly twice a week till he was 100 years old."

"Mrs. Jane Johnson, late of Leeds Workhouse, and

at present suffering temporary seclusion in the town gaol, is a living protest against the theory that excessive indulgence in alcoholic liquor tends to abbreviate the span of human existence. This vivacious old lady has attained the advanced age of 83, under circumstances which point to habitual intoxication as the leading incident in 'the story of her life from year to year.' On Wednesday morning she was brought up to the Leeds police-court for the two hundredth time, as she herself freely admitted, charged with being so helplessly drunk in the public streets that the executive were compelled to convey her to the lock-up in an ambulance."--*Daily Telegraph*.

William Thompson, of North Keyme, Lincolnshire, lived to 108.

"He smoked two pipes, and drank some ale, on the day of his death."

William Riddell, of Selkirk, in Scotland, died in 1718, aged 116.

This man was "remarkable for his love of brandy, which he drank in very large quantities. . . . He was not a drunkard (habitual), but he had frequent paroxysms of drinking, which continued several successive days. For the last two years of his life, his chief subsistence was a little bread infused in spirits and ale."

Pascal Seria, of Valentia, died at 111.

"Frequently smoked tobacco."

Richard Brown, of Peterchurch, Hereford, died in 1794, aged 108.

"In the instance of this old man, the assertion that smoking tobacco is prejudicial to health is completely refuted, as he was seldom seen without a pipe in his mouth, and took his last whiff a few hours before his death."

John Saunders, of Stratford, died in 1708, aged 106.

"He would walk to the Old Castle House, to drink a cup of ale and smoke his pipe."

John de la Somet, of Virginia, died in 1767, aged 130.

"He was a great smoker of tobacco, which, agreeing with his constitution, may not improbably be reckoned the cause of his uninterrupted health and longevity."

Joseph Creole, died in Caledonia, a little town of Wisconsin, on Jan. 27, 1866, aged 142.

"He was an inveterate smoker."

"Margaret Robertson, or Duncan, the oldest woman in Scotland, died at Coupar Angus, yesterday. She was born in 1773, and her husband, a weaver, died fifty years ago, and left her with a daughter, who is still alive, and over sixty. Mrs. Duncan was a *heavy smoker*, and until recently, when she became blind, was in possession of all her faculties. Her last illness was only of a week's duration."—*Daily Telegraph*, Sept. 17, 1879.

We do not advise either drinking or smoking, as a means of prolonging life; but still there is a philosophy noticed in the cases before us. Both drinking and smoking take away the appetite; less food is eaten,* therefore a less amount of earthy salts are taken into the system, and the cause of old age is delayed in its results; still sufficient food is taken to support life, and great age follows.

Total abstainers must not forget that alcohol is formed in their own bodies, and, as Sir B. Richardson says, "No man can be, in the strict scientific sense, a non-alcoholic, inasmuch as, 'will he, nill he,' he brews in his own economy 'a wee drap.' It is an innocent brew, certainly; but it is brewed, and the most ardent abstainer must excuse it. The fault, if it be one, rests with Nature, who, according to our poor estimates, is no more faultless than the rest of her sex."

Alcohol in excess is injurious to health, especially to the mental capabilities—the reasons of which will be entered upon hereafter. But there is no evidence to show that alcohol in moderation, and judiciously used, is detrimental to health.†

Tobacco affects the brain, the heart, circulation, and temperature. In excess it is therefore injurious.

* Alcohol by combining with oxygen, existing in the blood, becomes carbonic acid and water, thus reducing oxidation or waste of the system.

† We have experimented largely on the subject of alcohol, and can speak, to a certain extent, with authority. There is no doubt whatever that the habit of its excessive use is quickly acquired, especially by those who have a weak circulation, and to whom the added stimulus gives a feeling of cheerfulness and health. Persons of this temperament take to alcohol as a duck does to water. Shortly it becomes a truly nervous disease, for the simple reason that alcohol in excess is a solvent for phosphorus existing in an oxidisable form in the brain and nerves. We have heard temperance advocates ask the question,

Tobacco is, to a certain extent, a disinfectant: it mitigates the pangs of hunger, and soothes depression. How often it calms the temper! How many cross words are prevented in domestic life by the *moderate* use of tobacco!

Among other instances of longevity we have the Ancient Britons, whom Plutarch states "only began *to grow old* at 120 years."

"They were remarkable for their fine athletic form, for the great strength of their body, and for being swift of foot. They excelled in running, wrestling, climbing, and all kinds of bodily exercise; they were patient of pain, toil, and suffering of various kinds; were accustomed to fatigue, to bear hunger, cold, and all manner of hardships. They could run into morasses up to their necks, and live there for days without eating."—HENRY.

Boadicea, Queen of the Ancient Britons, in a speech to her army, when about to engage the degenerate Romans, said: "The great advantage we have over them is, that they cannot, like us, bear hunger, thirst, heat or cold; they must have fine bread, wine, and warm houses; to us every herb and

---

what is the natural drink of man? The general answer is *water*. The question itself, however, requires modification. Is it natural for man to drink? We say emphatically *no!* Adam did not drink in Eden at all, for the simple reason that his diet of luscious fruits ("fruits of the trees") contained both food and drink at the same time. Fruits contain from 80 to sometimes 95 per cent. of Nature's distilled water. The first inhabitants of Gan Eden did not thirst for liquid by itself—*they did not drink.*—*Vide Original Eden*, by the author.

root are food, every juice is our oil, and every stream of water our wine."

"Their arms, legs, and thighs were always left naked, and for the most part were painted blue. Their *food consisted almost exclusively of acorns, berries, and water.*"—GOLDSMITH.

From the above, we may justly infer that the Ancient Britons lived on a diet which contained comparatively a small amount of earthy salts; further, the acorn contains tanno-gallate of potash, which would harden the albuminous and gelatinous structures: they would therefore be less liable to waste and decay. Their endurance of hunger, cold, and hardships, and their love of water (probably from a hardened state of the skin), cannot be considered as mere fables.

Louisa Truxo, a negress, was stated to be living in June, 1780, at Cordova, in the Tucuman, South America, aged 175.

The council of the city took every means to verify the authenticity of this statement:

"On examination of the woman, it appeared that she perfectly remembered having seen the prelate Fernando Truxo, her first master, who died in the year 1614; and that a year before his death he gave *her*, together with other property, towards a fund for founding the university of that place. As no registers of baptism existed so long back, care was taken to collect every circumstance that could be brought forward in corroboration of the woman's statements. One of these proofs was the deposition of another female negro, named Manuela, who was known to be 120 years old, and she declared that, when she was quite a child, she remembered that Louisa Truxo was then an elderly woman."

Thomas Carn, according to the parish register of the church of St. Leonard, Shoreditch, died January 28, 1588, aged 207 years.

He is stated "to have been born in the reign of Richard II., A.D. 1381, and lived in the reigns of twelve kings and queens of England."

The *Petersburg Gazette* published, in 1812, an instance of a man, in the diocese of Ekaterinoslau, having attained an age of more than 200 years.

Spotswood, Archbishop of St. Andrews, says that Saint Mungo always slept on the bare ground, and attained the extraordinary age of 185 years.

Mr. Evans, of Spital Street, Spitalfields, died in 1730, aged 139, in complete possession of all his faculties. He well remembered the execution of Charles I., being seven years old at the time. Bailey, writing in 1855, says: "What a wonderful link does such a life form between the present and the past! There are, no doubt, numbers of persons still alive at this time who can well remember this remarkable old man. So that even the young men of this generation may be acquainted with individuals who knew the man who possibly witnessed an event which, at the present day, appears one of remote history."

"In the year 1566, a native of Bengal, named Numa de Cugna, died at the age of 370 years. He was a person of great simplicity, and quite illiterate, but of so extensive a memory that he was a kind of living chronicle, relating distinctly what had happened with his knowledge in the compass of his very long life, together with all the circumstances attending it."—MAFFEUS' *History of the Indies;* and confirmed by Ferdinand Costequedo, Historiographer Royal of Portugal.

Thomas Parr, a native of Shropshire, died in 1635, aged 152. He married at the age of eighty-eight, "seeming no older than many at forty."

He was brought to London by Thomas, then Earl of Arundel, to see Charles I., "when he fed high, drank plentifully of wines, by which his body was *overcharged*, his lungs obstructed, and the habit of the whole body quite disordered; in consequence, there could not but be speedy dissolution. If he had not changed his diet, he might have lived many years longer."—EASTON.

On his body being opened by Dr. Harvey, it was found to be in a most perfect state. "The heart was thick, fibrous, and fat; *his cartilages were not even ossified, as is the case in all old people,*" and the only cause to which death could be attributed was a "mere plethora, brought on by more luxurious living in London than he had been accustomed to in his native country, where his food was plain and homely."

In a poem by John Taylor, on the "old, old, very old man," the following outline of his diet is given:

> "He was of old Pythagoras' opinion,
> That green cheese was most wholesome with an *onion*,
> Coarse meslin bread, and for his daily swig,
> Milk, *buttermilk*, and water, *whey*, and whig.
> Sometimes metheglin, and for fortune happy,
> He sometimes supped a cup of ale most nappy."

He was married a second time at the age of a hundred and twenty-one, and could run in foot-races and perform the ordinary work of an agricultural labourer when 145 years old.

Henry Jenkins, of Ellerton, in Yorkshire, died in 1670, aged 169.

He remembered the battle of Flodden Field, in 1513, at which time he was twelve years of age. The registers of the Chancery and other courts prove that he gave evidence, and had an oath administered to him, 140 years before his death.

In the *Philosophical Transactions* of 1696, Sir Tancred Robinson states: "This Henry Jenkins, in the last century of his life, was a fisherman."

When ninety years of age, a child was born to him, and, when 160, he walked to London to have an audience with Charles II., and was able to swim across rapid rivers after he was 100. " His diet was coarse and *sour*."

Mrs. Clayton, of Springhead, died in 1867, aged 107 years.

"She was born in January, 1760. . . . Her health

was uniformly good; she generally rose at six in the morning, and retired at nine in the evening, and walked often to Gravesend, a distance of three miles, without apparent fatigue."

"A HEREFORDSHIRE CENTENARIAN.—On Monday Mrs. Webb, of Ledbury, widow of the late Mr. Thomas Webb, banker and deputy-lieutenant of Herefordshire, reached her hundredth birthday. She is the only surviving sister of the late Sir Joseph Thackwell, one of the heroes of Waterloo. Records in Berrow Church, near Ledbury, furnish proof. Mrs. Webb still enjoys good health, and she entertained a gathering of her relatives at her residence."
—*Standard*.

"There is now living at Copster Green, near Ribchester, a man named William Hayhurst, who has attained his hundredth and fourth year. On Tuesday a number of gentlemen gave a dinner in his honour. He was married, when twenty-six years of age, at Dinckley, near Whalley. He is very active yet; his hearing is good, but his eyesight is failing him. He has over thirty grandchildren and seventy great-grandchildren."—*Standard*.

"Another centenarian has been discovered. It appears that there is at present living in the Isle of Skye, a certain Widow Macpherson, who is approaching the close of the one hundred and sixth year of her age. She is, however, not a particularly interesting person, for though still blessed with a good memory, her experience and recollections lie within a very narrow and humble sphere. She has never been out of the island, nor does she understand a word of any language save Gaelic. The sanitary conditions under which she has lived are such as would be reckoned most pernicious by modern lecturers on health. Her home during the whole of her long life has been a turf hut of the most primitive construction, and yet she remembers six Lords of the Isles, nurtured in luxury and surrounded by plenty, who have followed each other to the grave in succession. She was born a few months after Johnson and Boswell paid their famous visit to the Isle of Skye, and the time that has elapsed since this has been one of the most remarkable epochs in the history of the world. Yet this illiterate islander can have been but very imperfectly acquainted with what was transpiring, and must have heard of the great events of her time in the form of vague rumours long out of date. What an interesting person she might have been had her long life been passed in the busy haunts of men, or in some centre of society! As it is, she can only be regarded as a physiological phenomenon, and a standing argument against the improvement of the dwellings of the Western Islanders. The turf hut is the lowest type of human habitation existing in this country, and it has puzzled visitors from our cities to know how it is possible for a person to remain, for even a few minutes, in the palpable reek, which rises from the peat-fire built in the centre of the floor, and fills the place to an apparently suffocating point, before it chooses to make its escape by the opening in the roof. Yet here we have a proof that it is not only possible to exist in such an atmosphere, but actually to prolong life to an age which has only on one or two occasions been reached in circumstances which are regarded as eminently favourable to longevity."—*Standard.*

"Constantinople is a tolerably ancient city, as European capitals go, but, old as it is, it never entertained within its gates since the date of its foundation a more remarkable visitor than the Circassian chieftain Hod Bey, who recently arrived in Stamboul, for the purpose of paying homage in person to his liege lord and hereditary commander, the Padishah. This warrior has attained an age which justifies him in regarding the venerable German Emperor as a mere stripling. He was born in 1762, and entered the Turkish military service in the year 1777, under the reign of Abdul Hamid I. Eight successive Sultans have known Hod Bey as one of the most faithful and valiant officers in the Ottoman Army, to which he still belongs, after an active military career of 105 years. He has fought in sixty-five pitched battles and innumerable skirmishes, received three-and-twenty wounds, and earned over and over again every war-decoration in the gift of the Grand Signior. Although well advanced in his hundred and twentieth year, he is strong and hearty, retains the use of all his faculties, and enjoys an excellent appetite. The present Sultan has shown him every attention that a sovereign can offer to a subject. No honour can be too great, no distinction too conspicuous, for a staunch old soldier who has fought for the Crescent throughout considerably more than a century."— *Daily Telegraph.*

Miguel Solis, of Bogota, San Salvador, who is supposed to be at least 180. At a congress of physicians, held at Bogota, Dr. Louis Hernandez read a report of his visit to this locally famous man, a country publican and farmer.

"We are told that he only confesses to this age (180 years); but his neighbours, who must be better able to judge, affirms that he is considerably older than he says. He is a half-bred, named Miguel Solis, and his existence is testified to by Dr. Hernandez, who was assured that when one of the 'oldest inhabitants' was a child, this man was recognised as a centenarian. His signature, in 1712, is said to have been discovered among those of persons who assisted in the construction of a certain convent (Franciscan convent at San Sebastian). Dr. Hernandez found this wonderful individual working in his garden. His skin was like parchment, his hair as white as snow, and covering his head like a turban. He attributed his long life to his careful habits; *eating only once a day,* for half an hour, because he believed that more food than could be eaten in half an hour could not be digested in twenty-four hours. He had been accustomed to *fast* on the first and fifteenth of every month, drinking, on those days, as *much water* as possible. He chose the most nourishing foods, and took all things cold."—*Lancet*, Sept. 7, 1878.

From this and other sources we gather the following habits of this man:

1. He eats but once a day, and only for half an hour.
2. He eats meat but twice a month; from which we may justly infer that he is to a certain extent abstemious in his daily meal.
3. He drinks large quantities of water.
4. He fasts two whole days every month.

From these habits it follows that, compared with the majority of mankind, he eats little, yet enough to support life; he therefore takes into his system a small amount of earthy compounds, which therefore take a longer period to accumulate, and produce the symptoms of decrepitude and old age at a far later period than they occur in most individuals who live upon an ordinary quantity of food, whose bodies become rigid, decrepit, and ossified, we will say, at about "three-score years and ten." Further, that his drinking large quantities of water, which, if not unusually hard, will tend to dissolve and remove those earthy compounds, which are not the *effect* but the *cause* of old age. We have not thought it necessary to make further inquiries concerning the diet and habits of this man. Our information is derived from numerous periodicals, and we only arrive at the above conclusions because we are convinced, from ascertained facts and experiments, that man may by diet alone attain the age which Miguel Solis is supposed to be.

As another instance of longevity, we must not omit to mention Sir Moses Montefiore—"one of the best and worthiest of God's missionaries to all mankind." His hundredth birthday was celebrated at Ramsgate on Oct. 28th, 1884.

A man named Henry Leadville has just died at Grand Bassa, Liberia, at the reputed age of 129 years. He was born in Missouri, and emigrated from there to Liberia in 1889. He settled at a place called Fortsville, and was known to the people as "Uncle Henry." The old man became possessed of one of the finest country seats in the rural district of Grand Bassa, and just before his death had the pleasure of gathering the first crop of coffee from trees which he had planted when he first settled in Liberia, in the spring of 1889.—*People*, Nov. 1894.

Besides longevity, we notice in Nature a power of restoration, which will be seen from the following cases :

Philip Laroque, to whom we have before referred—

"At the age of ninety-two, cut *four large teeth*."

A Mr. Mazarella, of Vienna, died in 1774, aged 105.

"A few months before his death he had *several new teeth*; and his *hair*, grown grey by age, *became black*, its original colour."

Numa de Cugna, the Bengalese tercentenarian before referred to—

"Had *four new sets of teeth*; and the colour of his

hair and beard had been frequently changed from black to grey, and from grey to black."

Lord Bacon says the Countess of Desmond, who lived to 148, *renewed her teeth* once or twice.

Mary How, of Mapleton, Derby, died in 1751, from the effects of a fall from an apple-tree, aged 112.

"Two years before her death she *cut several new teeth*, and her *hair changed its colour.*"

Lady Angélique Domenqieux de Sempe, of Noniliac, in France, died in 1759, aged 103.

She "had *several new teeth* when near ninety years of age."

Susan Edmonds, of Winterbourne, Hants, died in 1780, aged 104.

"Five years before her death she had *new hair*, of a fine brown colour, which began to turn grey a few months before her death.

Sarah Williams, of Brent Tor, near Tavistock, died in 1809, aged 108."

"When in about her hundredth year, she cut *five new teeth.*"

Elizabeth Spencer, widow, died in 1806, aged 105.

"For many years she was entirely deprived of sight; but about her one hundredth year she *recovered the use of her eyes*, which continued with her till the close of her life."

Janet Allan, of Kilmarnock, Ayrshire, died in 1788, aged 105 years.

"Four years before her death, her *sight*, which for long had been dim, in a great measure **returned**, so that she could see much better than had been the case for a number of years."

Owen Duffy, of Monaghan county, Ireland.

The *Dublin Freeman* of July 29, 1854, stated that this individual was then alive, aged 122 years. Having lost his second wife when he was 116, he married a third, a young woman, by whom he had a *son* and a *daughter*. At this time his youngest son was two years old, whilst his eldest was ninety.

Mrs. Jane Lewson, widow, of No. 12, Coldbath Square, London, died in 1816, aged 116.

She was left in affluent circumstances. Her apartments were never washed, her windows never cleaned, and she never practised ablutions of any kind whatever, for fear of taking cold. She "cut *two new teeth* at the age of eighty-seven."

Margaret Melvil, of Kettle, Fifeshire, died in 1783, aged 117.

"She *renewed several teeth* at a hundred years of age."

Marian Gibson, of Galston, died at 100.

"When she was about ninety years of age, she had a *new set of teeth*."

Rebecca Poney, of the Poor-house, Norton Folgate, lived to 106.

"She cut *two new teeth* at the age of 102."

John Weeks, of New London, Connecticut, died at 114.

When he was 106, he married a girl of sixteen, at which time "his grey hairs had fallen off, which were renewed by a *dark* head of *hair;* and several *new teeth* made their appearance."

"John Rousey, Esq., of the island of Distey, in Scotland, died in 1738, aged 137.

"He had a *son* at *one hundred* years of age, who inherited his estate."

John Riva, of Venice, died at 116.

"He always chewed citron-bark, and had a child after he was 100."

Margaret Krasiona, of the village of Koninia, in Poland. When ninety-four years of age, she married her third husband, who was then 105.

"They lived together fourteen years, and had two boys and one girl. This is certified in the parish registers of the village of Ciwousin, district of Stensick, in the palatine of Sendomir.

Thomas Parr, when 102 years old, had a child by Catherine Milton, for which he did penance.

Dr. Stare states that his grandfather, a native of Bedfordshire, and who died in his hundredth year, "at the age of eighty-five, had a *complete set of new teeth;* and his *hair*, from being of a snowy white, gradually *became darker."—Philosophical Transactions*, vol. xxiii.

"A magistrate named Bauborg, who lived at Rochingen, in the Palatinate, and who died in 1791, in the hundred and twentieth year of his age. In 1787, long after he had lost all his *teeth*, eight *new* ones *grew up*. At the end of six months they again dropped out, but their place was supplied by other new ones, both in the upper and the lower jaw; and nature, unwearied, continued this labour for years, and even till within a month of his death. After he had employed his new teeth for some time with great convenience in chewing his food, they took their leave, and new ones immediately sprang up in some of their sockets. All these teeth he acquired and lost without any pain; and the whole number of them amounted at least to fifty."—HUFELAND.

"The *Auxilia Breton* mentions a curious circumstance. It states that a gendarme named Labe, of the Department of the Ille et Vilaine, who had a grey beard and hair, presented himself a few days ago perfectly black! He said he had had a *determination of blood to the head*, which caused his head to swell and become black, as did also his beard and hair and part of his body. He had felt great pain for a time, but that afterwards he found himself much better; that then his skin resumed its natural colour, but that the hair and beard *remained black*.* Two comrades of the gendarme, one of them a corporal, confirmed his statements."—*Morning Advertiser*.

A patient of the author's, sixty-one years of age, living in First Street, Chelsea, cut three new teeth in 1878.

* "In my work on 'Healthy Skin,' I have mentioned several instances of very old persons in whom the natural colour of the hair returned after they had been for years before grey. This was the case with John Weeks, who lived to the age of 114. Sir John Sinclair reports a similar occurrence in an old Scotchman, who lived to be 110; and Susan Edmonds, when in her 95th year, recovered her black hair, but became again grey previously to her death at the age of 105."—SIR ERASMUS WILSON.

"By an inscription on a tombstone at Breslau, it appears that one John Montanus, who was a dean there, recovered three times the colour of his hair. . . . Does it therefore appear incredible or impossible that man may occasionally after his 'three score and ten,' again exhibit the powers and physical qualities of youth?"

A few years ago the *Times* gave an account of a lady more than eighty years of age, who cut her *third set of teeth*, and whose features were said to have the *juvenescence of thirty years.*

The above-mentioned cases are but a few of many which have been collected. We cannot therefore consider such changes impossible; Nature has repeatedly accomplished them, apparently by accident; but what Nature accomplishes apparently by accident, may become a possibility, if we are able to discover the laws and principles which govern such changes, and if we are further able to apply them and regulate their action.

In the animal kingdom we find numerous cases of longevity: the first we notice is in reptiles, which are cold-blooded, with slight powers of respiration, and whose internal and external consumption is therefore much less than in warm-blooded animals. They are very tenacious of life, and most of them have a power of reproducing and restoring destroyed organs; thus earthworms restore themselves after being cut with a spade; the head and horns of a snail will grow again in six months: the limbs and tail of a water-newt are replaced in a few months, and even if its eye is destroyed, another is perfected in about ten months.

"A toad was found at Organ, in France, in a well which had been covered up for 150 years. It was torpid, but revived on being exposed. Many well-authenticated cases are recorded of toads found alive in old stones and in old trees, where they must have lived for many centuries."—SIR RICHARD PHILLIPS.

The *Transactions of the Swedish Academy* give an account of a toad found in 1733 in a stone quarry, seven ells deep, in the middle of a hard block of stone, and which was extricated with much labour by hammer and chisel, and was alive, though very weak. Its skin is described as being shrivelled, "covered here and there with a stony crust."

"A STRANGE DISCOVERY.—A strange discovery was made in the De Beers Mine recently. Two diamonds were found embedded in a piece of well-preserved wood, found at a depth of 700 feet. On splitting the block, which was fully ten inches thick, a cavity was disclosed to view in which reposed a living specimen of a tree frog. The local scientific people compute the age of the tree at 180 years, during 150 of which froggy had been entombed. The jumping creature did not, however, long survive the shock of gazing upon a busy world, after so long a seclusion, but soon expired. Figuratively speaking, it lives—in a phial of spirit—at the Kimberley Museum. At different times curious articles have been found in exploitation for diamonds, but the most interesting discoveries lately are the skeletons of a remarkably tall race of men, primitive mining tools, etc., which have been recovered from old diamond mines in the Free State. Everything seems to show that these mines were extensively worked, but by what race the natives of the region have not even a tradition."—*Nov.*, 1894.

"The *testudo* or tortoise is so long-lived that two are recorded in England which lived 120 and 200 years. . . . In the library of Lambeth Palace is the shell of a tortoise, brought there in 1623. It lived till 1730, and was then accidentally killed. Another in the palace at Fulham, procured by Bishop Laud in 1628, died in 1753. One at Peterborough lived 220 years."—SIR R. PHILLIPS.

The crocodile and alligator, which many travellers assert increase in size as long as they exist, from what is at present known, seem to live to very great ages.

Serpents live to almost incredible ages, and many believe they never die from " natural causes."

"When it (the serpent) is old, by squeezing itself between two rocks, it can strip off its old skin, and so grows *young again*."—CALMET'S *Dictionary*.

"Snakes, frogs, lizards, etc., cast their skin every year; and it appears that this method of becoming again young contributes very much to their support and duration."—HUFELAND.

Many reptiles cast their skins; this is especially noticed in snakes. In casting its skin a large quantity of gelatinous and earthy matter, which by its accumulation has gradually given rise to the characteristics of "old age," is thrown off; the animal is relieved of them, and becomes in the full sense of the term young again. There may, therefore, be a profound philosophy in the command. "Be ye therefore *wise as serpents* and harmless as doves."

Crabs and lobsters undergo a rejuvenescence in casting their shells annually; and for about four days they are naked and defenceless. Their size increases only when in this soft state; their mail, which contains a large quantity of earthy matter, soon prevents further expansion until it is cast off, when the animal is again allowed to increase in size.

In fishes many instances of extraordinary longevity are recorded, which is especially marked in those of slow growth.

"Carp grow but two or three inches *per annum*, and live to a great age; some in the lake at Fontainebleau being two or three hundred years old . . . Whales live many centuries."—*Million of Facts.*

"We know from the ancient Roman history, that in the imperial fish-ponds there were several lampreys (murænæ) which had attained to their sixtieth year; and which had at length become so well acquainted and familiar with man, that *Crassus, orator, unam ex illis defleverit.*"*—HUFELAND.

"The pike, a dry, exceedingly voracious animal, and carp also, according to undeniable testimony,

* That Crassus, the orator, shed tears for one of them when it died.

prolong their life to 150 years, The salmon grows rapidly and dies soon. On the other hand, the perch, the growth of which is slower, preserves its existence longer."—HUFELAND.

"Gesner says that the longevity of the pike is almost incredible; he mentions as an instance one that was taken in Hailborn, in Swabia, in the year 1497, with these words engraven on a ring: 'I am the fish that was first of all put into this lake by Frederick Second, Oct. 5th, 1230.' This gave it the age of two hundred and sixty-seven years."— RHIND'S *Six Days of Creation*.

"Some species of fish and certain snakes are said to live till some accident puts an end to their *indefinite term of life*."—SOUTHEY.

In birds a renovation is noticed in the process of moulting, during which the old feathers are cast off, and with them fibrinous, gelatinous and earthy substances, and new feathers are acquired, which, by their growth, remove certain quantities of these solid substances from the system.

Many cases of longevity are recorded in birds, especially those which live on fruits, fish, and other animal foods.

It is affirmed that some of the parrot species live in their natural state to "ages ranging from five to seven hundred years."

"One has instances of its living sixty years a prisoner with man, and how old may it not have been when it was caught?"

"The swan lives 200 years;" some authorities even prolong this to 300.

"Some time ago, a male swan, which had seen many generations come and go, and witnessed the other mutations incidental to the lapse of 200 years, died at Rosemount. He was brought to Dunn when the late John Erskine, Esq., was in his infancy, and was then said to be 100 years old. About two years ago he was purchased by the late David Duncan, Esq., of Rosemount, and within that period his mate brought him forth four young ones, which he destroyed as soon as they took the water. Mr. Mallison Bridget (in whose museum the bird is now to be seen) thinks it might have lived much longer but for a lump or excrescence at the top of the windpipe, which, on dissecting him, he found to be composed of grass and tow. This is the same bird that was known and recognised in the early years of octogenarians, in this and the neighbouring parishes, by the name of the 'Old Swan of Dunn.'"—*Medical Gazette.*

In 1782 "Farmer Pope, of Beaminster, Dorset, had a goose eighty-six years old, which had been on the farm with four successive tenants."

The raven, rook, crow, hawk, seagull, pelican, heron, crane, and other birds of a similar nature, are believed to live beyond a hundred years.

According to the *Eleveur*, many birds, such as the eagle, the swan, and the raven, live more than a hundred years. The parrot, the heron, the goose, and the pelican have been known to live for sixty years; the peacock for 25 years, the pigeon 20, the crane 20, the linnet 25, the goldfinch 15, the lark 13, the blackbird 12, the canary 24, the pheasant 15, the thrush 10, the cock 10, the robin redbreast 12, and the wren only 3 years.

The inferior animals, which live, in general, regular and temperate lives, have generally their prescribed term of years. The horse lives twenty-five years, the ox fifteen or twenty, the lion about twenty, the dog ten or twelve, the rabbit eight, the guinea-pig six or seven years. These numbers all bear a similar proportion to the time the animal takes to grow its full size. But man, of all the animals, is the one that seldom comes up to his average. He ought to live one hundred years, according to this physiological law, for five times twenty are one hundred; but, instead of that, he scarcely reaches, on the average, four times his growing period, the cat six times, and the rabbit even eight times the standard of measurement. The reason is obvious—man is not only the most irregular and the most intemperate, but the most laborious and hard-worked of all the animals.

Tacitus says the eagle lives to 500 years, and there are instances of its having lived in confinement more than 100, and one died at Vienna aged 104.

"A gentleman at London a few years ago received from the Cape of Good Hope one (a falcon) that had been caught with a golden collar, on which was inscribed, in English, 'His Majesty K. James of England. An. 1610.' It had therefore been at liberty 182 years from the time of its escape. How old was it when it escaped? It was of the largest species of these birds, and possessed still no little strength and spirit; but it was remarked that its eyes were blind and dim, and that the feathers of its neck had become white."—HUFELAND.

In the *mammalia* the elephant perhaps attains the greatest age.

"They grow for thirty or forty years, and live 200 or 300; some say 400 years."

An elephant called Hannibal died in 1859, in a travelling circus in America. "He was extremely old. We have heard his age stated variously at from 500 to 1000 years."[*]

After Alexander the Great had vanquished Porus, King of India, he took a large elephant which had fought valiantly in battle for the king, and called him Ajax, dedicating him to the sun, and setting him free with the following inscription:

"Alexander, the sun of Jupiter, hath dedicated Ajax to the sun."

This elephant was found 350 years afterwards with the inscription.

Speaking of the longevity of the elephant, Thomson says:

> "With gentle might endued,
> Though powerful, yet not destructive; here he sees
> Revolving ages sweep the changeful earth,
> And empires rise and fall; regardless he
> Of what the never-resting race of man project."

[*] *Reynolds' Miscellany.*

INSTANCES OF LONGEVITY.

Elephants "live on vegetables," and in their natural state are very fond of the young and tender shoots and leaves of trees; their diet is therefore one adapted to longevity. Moreover, the tusk or tooth "weighs from 120 to 200 lbs.," and one hundred parts contain twenty-four of gelatine and sixty-four of carbonate of lime; the tusks therefore relieve the system of an elephant of from nearly 80 to 128 lbs. of lime; these are furthermore *cast*, being found in the woods of Africa and Ceylon, but how often and at how long a period is as yet undetermined.

The wild hog lives chiefly on roots, and is said to live in its native state "to the age of 300 years."

A "lion lived seventy years in the Tower;" we may therefore justly infer, that in its natural state it lives beyond a century.

The camel "generally attains the age of fifty, and sometimes of 100 years." "It eats *little* and drinks less."

"They require *little* and coarse food, and live for ten or fifteen days without water."

The horse in its wild state lives to upwards of fifty years; but when brought to subjugation by the severity of man, he seldom attains half this age.

It is a well-known fact that when a horse does little work, and passes the greater part of his days—especially the early ones—in his pasture, he lives to nearly forty years; but when a horse is hard worked, and the process of transpiration thereby increased, and is, moreover, fed upon beans, oats, and other "ossifying" foods, his days are much shorter; few, in fact, reach twenty years, and even "Eclipse," a race-horse which for speed is said to have never been defeated, with all the attention man could bestow, died at twenty-five years.

This faithful servant of man soon becomes prematurely old from the diet on which he is fed; in fact, his food contains so much earthy matter that concretions *(hippolithi)* of phosphates of lime, magnesia, and ammonium, in the cæcum are of very common occurrence; the deposition of earthy salts in the system is also accelerated by hard work, which increases the process of transpiration.

From the above few cases of the ages of reptiles, birds, and animals, which we have selected as illustrations, it is clear that those of them which attain the greatest longevity in animated nature are those which are subject to or possessed of one or more of the following peculiarities or qualities:

1. Those which are only slightly susceptible to the action of atmospheric *oxygen*.

2. Those which are possessed of a *restorative* power, or are enabled to throw off from the system fibrinous, gelatinous, and earthy matter; and the more perfect this renovation, the greater the duration of life.

3. Those which subsist upon food which contains a small quantity of earthy compounds.

4. Those which eat but little or seldom.

In the vegetable kingdom are numerous instances of longevity.

INSTANCES OF LONGEVITY.

"A lime in the Grisons is fifty-one feet round and about 600 years old."

"A dragon's-blood tree in Teneriffe was forty-eight feet round and 1,000 years old."

"The *cubbeer burr*, near Baroach, has 350 main trunks and 3,000 small ones. It is believed to be 3,000 years old."

One specimen of the African *baobab* was estimated by its circles to be 5,700 years old by Adanson and Humboldt.

Adanson found some of these trees only six feet in diameter, with the names of seafaring men who visited them in the fifteenth and sixteenth centuries cut on them, and with the incisions little extended.

There is a cypress in Mexico 120 feet round, which De Canolle considers older than Adanson's baobab.

The yew attains great age; those "at Fountain's Abbey are about 1,200 years old;" one "at Crowhurst 1,500;" one at Fortingal above 2,000 years; and one at Braburn, the age of which is stated to be from 2,500 to 3,000 years.

"A chestnut in Gloucestershire is 900, and one at Saucerre 600 years."

"Terebinth-trees, the El-Elah of the Bible, live 1,500 or 2,000 years, but neglect has rendered them scarce in Syria."

A chestnut was planted in 800 at Tamworth; it was a boundary called the "Great Chestnut-tree" in the reign of Stephen, in 1135, and "in 1759 it bore nuts, which produced young trees;" and it was stated to be fifty-two feet round.

"Two orange-trees at Rome, planted by St. Dominic and Thomas Aquinas, are from 500 to 600 years old."

An apple-tree was stated to be in existence in 1820 at Woolstrope, "from which Newton saw an apple fall in 1665."

Ivies have been recorded which have lived five hundred years, and the elm, larch, and other trees are stated to live the same or even a longer period.

The oak is slow of growth and reaches a great age. De Canolle states that there are oaks in France 1,500 years old. The Wallace oak, near Paisley, is more than 700 years old.

"Some olives, near Jerusalem, are 800 years old."

Throughout the animal and vegetable kingdoms, with a few exceptions, which would be too lengthy to enter upon in the present work, a similar cause of natural death is observed to that which we have traced to man; and even the stately and venerable oak, which inspires us with reverence and awe, when we contemplate that the tree we gaze upon perhaps once shaded our wild ancestors and the Druids, only dies because the central and oldest parts of the wood gradually acquire such compactness, hardness, and want of porosity, that it becomes incapable of imbibing or receiving further nourishment; a process analogous to "induration" and "ossification" in man and animals.

CHAPTER V.

THE PREVENTION OF DISEASE.

AS the majority of mankind die unnatural deaths, from disease or accident, most of them being the result of either ignorance or carelessness, we feel it a duty to draw attention to some of the attributes of civilization which so largely tend to cause unnecessary disease and premature death.

Sanitary science is now so popular, that we will commence this chapter with a few remarks on the best methods of domestic sanitation.

In the majority of old houses the drainage system will be found so sadly deficient in scientific principle, that the only wonder is that, as a people, we remain as healthy as we are. It is thus hardly necessary to point out the vast importance of this social problem to the welfare of the community.

As the subject is so surrounded with technicalities, we must content ourselves with giving a few general rules:

1. Drain-pipes passing through a house should in all cases be surrounded with concrete, but the best systems place all drain-pipes as much as possible outside the building. All pipes used for house-drains should be glazed and non-porous.

2. Waste and overflow-pipes should be ventilated to the outer air before reaching the main sewer.

3. The pipes supplying water and gas should on no account be laid in the same trench with the drain-pipes; their course should be as much above ground as possible, as they require frequent attention.

4. Closets should never be built in the centre of a house. They should invariably be provided with a window opening into the outer air. They should not be supplied with water from the same cistern which contains the water used for drinking purposes.

5. Cisterns should be cleansed frequently.

6. It is most unwise to become the tenant of a house without first consulting some competent authority as to its sanitary arrangements.

Ventilation.—Draughts must be avoided, as they frequently are the cause of cold, inflammation of the lungs, and numerous other diseases. The common idea that the noxious character of confined air is due to a deficiency of oxygen is erroneous. A slight deficiency of oxygen, if counterbalanced merely by a similar increase in the amount of nitrogen, is not injurious to man.

But those gases (chiefly carbonic acid) which are produced in close and confined rooms and workshops are the immediate cause, by their poisonous influence on the blood, of that stagnating sub-oxidation which gradually lays the foundation of many wasting diseases.

The inhalation of carbonic acid, even in comparatively small quantities, in the atmosphere, causes the white corpuscles of the blood to enlarge, and thus to become less capable of circulation. Independent of this action, the interchange between atmospheric oxygen and the carbonic acid formed in the system is decreased, and morbid and definite products are formed in the blood. A septic condition is subsequently set up in that portion of the system most exposed to the atmosphere—viz., the lungs, the tissues of which become oxidised and undergo a semi-decomposition, thus producing *bacilli*, which in *primary* consumption are a result and not a cause of the disease. These *bacilli*, moreover, under certain conditions, have the power of causing the same action in substances capable of the same changes—*i.e.*, if a person in delicate health or predisposed to consumption inhales the breath or dried sputa of a consumptive patient, *bacilli* may be introduced into the lungs, and thus be in one person the cause of the disease, though in the first patient they were but the result.

Polluted air is productive of much more general injury than impure water. The air of rooms in which human beings live or sleep ought to be in a constant state of motion, but not sufficiently to produce a draught.

As hot air ascends, there should be in ordinary sized rooms several outlets near the ceiling for the egress of impure air, and a similar number of inlets near the floor for the introduction of fresh air. A few holes bored in the lower part of the window-sash and in the upper part of the door will answer the purpose.

A trumpet-mouthed tube (like a penny toy-trumpet) inserted in the holes in the lower sash of the upper division of the window will assist in diffusing the fresh air so admitted.

No one should sleep in a room which has been inhabited during the day, unless the windows have been kept open and an interchange of air allowed.

In large houses the staircase is often the means of accumulating vitiated air in the upper rooms. It is, therefore, necessary that a proper ventilator should *be placed in the roof over the highest landing-place.*

The average temperature of a house should be kept at about 67° Fahr., and the best means of providing artificial warmth is by a system of hot-water pipes.

Gas.—This method of lighting, though highly useful in the public streets, is very prejudicial to health when used in private rooms, the products of its combustion being more injurious vapours than those produced by burning candles or lamps. Concert-rooms, theatres, and other public halls, and even the living-rooms of ordinary houses, often become much overheated from the use of gas. On quitting them for the outer air, there is great danger that the sudden change may produce cold, and in some cases even lay the foundation of pulmonary disease.

The use of the electric light is a move in the right direction. The latest improved electric lamps produce neither heat nor deleterious gas, and the sooner they supplant the ordinary methods of lighting in private houses the better. Gas should on no account be burnt in sleeping apartments during the night.

Cleanliness.—Although numerous individuals have attained great ages without much attention to personal cleanliness, it is nevertheless certain that a clean skin, clean clothing, and clean rooms tend more to the preservation of health than all the more advanced sciences combined. The skin is an organ, the importance of which cannot be over-estimated. There are about 2,800 pores or outlets of the sweat-glands to the square inch, and the total length of these little tubes would cover a distance of twenty-eight miles. It is superfluous to point out the evil results which accrue when these outlets become clogged. Judicious bathing tends not only to cleanliness, but is eminently strengthening. For those in fair health a cold bath each morning will be found a great safeguard against taking cold, and an invigorating practice. The skin should afterwards be well rubbed with a rough towel.

For those in delicate health a tepid bath is preferable, but the rubbing should not be forgotten.

A warm bath, with soap, should of course be taken weekly, or oftener.

Sea bathing is beneficial to many persons, but does not suit all constitutions. Never bathe on a full stomach, or when exhausted from fatigue. The majority of persons remain in the water too long. Fifteen minutes should be the maximum.

Exercise.—There is no greater preservative of health than regular exercise. Of all exercises that of walking is the very best. A brisk walk of three or four miles should never be omitted by those who desire to enjoy sound health, unless their means admit of horse exercise. In the absence of the latter, the fashionable pastime of "cycling," if not pushed beyond reasonable limits, is beneficial and exhilarating. Of outdoor games, of course all depends upon age, strength, habits, etc.; but for ladies, and even those of the sterner sex, who have passed the meridian, lawn tennis forms an attractive and healthful pursuit. Excessive and fatiguing exercise is doubtless ultimately productive of serious injury to the system. We would advise all who are fond of violent exercise to be moderate, and to seek variety.

Drilling and gymnastics are beneficial to boys at school.

One of the great objects of exercise is to equalize the circulation, thus preventing congestions, especially those of the liver, which are the prevailing characteristic of the present generation. The circulation of the blood through the arteries and capillaries is one of the means whereby the frame is nourished and supported, and the organs of digestion strengthened. Thus sufficient exercise will not only improve the health, spirits, and physical powers, but will render such things as tonics and alteratives unnecessary.

Change of Air.—For invalids a change of air from one room to another is better than no change at all. It is unnecessary to point out the benefits of a few weeks in the country or at the seaside, at suitable intervals, especially for brain-workers and delicate females.*

* The system of treatment where a tendency to consumption exists, advocated by Dr. J. Hartnett, by which the air is thoroughly impregnated with volatile antiseptics, is the most rational yet advocated for the cure of pulmonary consumption. The apparatus in use is

Sleep.—Too much stress cannot be laid on the absolute necessity of sufficient sleep; also, that rest must be taken at the proper time.

The electric and atmospheric conditions are entirely different in the daytime, and no amount of sleep during daylight is of the same benefit as a good night's rest. Seven or eight hours' sleep is necessary for the equalization of the circulation, the rest and recuperation of the body, and the proper nourishment of the brain.

Late suppers are injurious; but some individuals are, from habit, so peculiarly constituted as to be unable to sleep on an empty stomach. These persons should partake of some light refreshment about two hours before retiring to rest.

Luxury in sleeping accessories should be avoided. Hair or wool mattresses are infinitely more healthful

worked by electricity. The air is thoroughly filtered and dried and charged to the fullest extent with Alpine Pine, Tasmanian Euculyptus, and other preparations. The result is that an atmosphere resembling mountain and Pine Forest air, in its purity and fragrance, is produced. The effect of this on the lungs is that the bacteria of consumption, the bacilli, are killed, and their excreta, the toxines or poisons which produce the distressing symptoms, are destroyed. The system of respiratory gymnastics, advocated by the same author in his work on the *Antiseptic Inhalation Cure of Consumption*, is undoubtedly rational in the extreme. The chest walls are thoroughly expanded, and a greater amount of surface exposed to the action of the antiseptic dry air, and a freer ventilation of the lungs takes place than during ordinary respiration. Both those systems combined cause the expulsion from the system of the living parasites, which undoubtedly cause the disease. The system of using an apparatus in the sleeping rooms of patients, and even healthy individuals, by which the air is kept in a pure antiseptic condition throughout the night, is undoubtedly a great preventative against consumption and other infectious diseases.

than feather beds, and the lighter the bedclothing the better.

Clothing.—Nothing is more necessary to a comfortable and congenial state of existence than that the body should be kept at as nearly as possible a uniform temperature.

Any degree of cold which produces shivering cannot be endured without injury to health. The purpose of clothing is to prevent the loss of bodily heat by radiation. Wool, being a better non-condutor of heat, is a better substance for clothing than silk or cotton, and the more loose and easy the fit, the more warmth will the garment afford, because a stratum of warm air is allowed to interpose between it and the body.

Tight clothing, including stays, is dangerous, both by its action in arresting circulation and producing deformity, and by its tendencey to confine the movements of the external limbs and cramp natural actions of the internal organs.

Flannels worn during the winter should not be too suddenly cast off. Merino, however, forms a good substitute during the excessive heat.

The action of oxygen upon some of the constituents of the blood and tissues of the body is one of the sources of animal heat. The skin, by increase of perspiration, and its evaporation, carries off the excess, so that the internal parts of the body are, in health, preserved at a uniform temperature of about 98·2°. The excretory function of the skin is of paramount importance in regard to health.

THE PREVENTION OF DISEASE.

A diminution of the insensible perspiration is a characteristic of many diseases and a concomitant of most fevers.

If a man be exposed to a cold temperature (say 40°), his skin becomes almost insensible, and the vessels which *supply* the perspiration contract, and perspiration ceases. Again, under a very hot temperature, perspiration is increased—its evaporation producing cold. Thus an almost even temperature is kept up. How necessary, therefore, is it, that in winter we should be clad in warm garments to keep off the cold influence of the external air, and that in summer we should be clad in garments which, instead of absorbing heat, refract it, and allow free ventilation and evaporation to the skin.

In this climate many persons wear nearly the same amount of clothing during the winter and summer. For this reason, in the hot days of summer, which, during the season just passed (1884) have approached tropical heat, the excessive temperature was felt even more severely than in the tropics, where loose and thin cotton garments are worn. It is absurd, in this changeable climate, to be guided by the seasons. In a cold summer an overcoat will often be found of more comfort than in a warm winter, as the temperature of December has been known to be higher than that of August in the same year. Changes should therefore be carefully watched, and the dress altered accordingly.

Infant Rearing.—It is astonishing to witness the amount of ignorance on this point amongst mothers —especially young ones. It is the duty of a mother to hand down her experiences to her daughter, even during the childhood of the latter, in order that when she grows up she may know distinctly and thoroughly how to rear her own offspring. It is of paramouut importance, and also a bounden duty of the nation, not only to encourage the study of the subject, but to make it compulsory that the simple laws and duties relating to the rearing of infant humanity should be taught to the elder girls in all our schools. We have already shown in a previous chapter that *human* milk is the best adapted to infant life, and have given the chemical and physiological reasons for the statement. The next best food for infants is asses' milk, which is, however, an expensive commodity. The majority of mothers use *cows' milk* diluted with about one-third its bulk of water. It is better to add a little sugar.

The bottle and tube should be cleansed daily, or oftener ; and if any of the residue be found to be at all sour, the bottle should be carefully washed with warm water, to which a little soda has been added.

No other food but milk, diluted as above, is required, and a child may take from two to three pints daily. The prevalent custom of giving lime-water in milk to children is unnecessary, and frequently leads to premature ossification of the child, thus stunting its growth. Cows' milk contains quite enough lime for the formation of the bones and teeth. We are now speaking of healthy children; but if a child suffers from rickets, which results from the solvent action of certain acids formed in its own blood—not from a deficiency of phosphates in the food—the lime should be given as a phosphate, or better still, as a hypophosphite.

If a child is brought up partly by the breast and partly by hand, the mixture of human and cows' milk is not deleterious. The popular prejudice of nurses on this point is fallacious.

Many foods, including "tops and bottoms" biscuits, boiled bread, etc., are not adapted as a diet for children under seven months old. After that age, some farinaceous food is desirable, of which there are numerous suitable preparations. After twelve months a little broth, gravy, or eggs may be added.

About the third year a little meat may also be given, and at eight or nine the ordinary diet of the family may be partaken of. Up to this age milk should form one of the most important articles of diet.

In regard to marriage, we have only to state that nearly all persons who have attained remarkable longevity were married. Marriage, as Hufeland states, "tends to moderate overstrained hope and enthusiastic speculation, as well as excessive care. Everything, by the participation of another being— by the intimate connexion of our existence with that of another—is rendered milder and more supportable."

Independently of the physical education of children, their mental training should not be neglected, but a child should not begin to learn too soon. We constantly witness the bad effects of too early and excessive mental application, which induces imperfectly formed limbs, round shoulders, muscular weakness, and narrow chests, from the confined and unnatural sitting postures in which children at a young age are kept, sometimes for hours, at school. At the age of puberty, great care should be taken of both sexes, and a heavy responsibility rests upon parents. Girls should be instructed in the ways of modesty, cleanliness, and health. Boys should be warned of the evil consequences of anything unnatural, from which many evils arise, in order that, morally, mentally, and physically, they may lay the foundation of a long and healthful life.

Had we really prudent and far-seeing parents at the present time, we might hope for young men such as are described by the ancient poet Bürger, in the following lines:

> "He who in Pleasure's downy arms
> Ne'er lost his health or youthful charms,
> A hero lives ; and justly can
> Exclaim, 'In me behold a man !'

> "He prospers like the slender reed,
> Whose top waves gentle o'er the mead ;
> And moves, such blessings virtue follow,
> In health and beauty an Apollo.

> "So full of majesty, a god,
> Shall earth alone be his abode?
> With dignity he steps, he stands,
> And nothing fears ; for he commands.

> "Like drops drawn from the crystal stream
> His eyes with pearly brilliance beam ;
> With blushing signs of health o'erspread,
> His cheeks surpass the morning's red.

> "The fairest of the female train
> For him shall bloom, nor bloom in vain.
> O happy she whose lips he presses !
> O happy she whom he caresses !"

CHAPTER VI.

AGENTS BEST ADAPTED FOR A LENGTHENED PROLONGATION OF EXISTENCE.

BY the term *agents* best adapted to prolong life we mean those substances or compounds which, by their action in or upon the system, tend to check the *cause* of "old age" and "natural death," and which tend to prevent or even remove the accumulations which we have already shown are not the *effect*, but the *cause*, of the changes which are observed as age advances, either by preventing the excessive action of atmospheric *oxygen*; or by removing *earthy* compounds, which have accumulated to an extent more than is requisite to supply the wants of the system; or those substances which combine the two actions.

To commence with *solvents*, or those agents which tend to prevent the accumulation of earthy matter in the system, the first we notice is *water*.

When water is decomposed by electricity, the hydrogen at the negative pole is double the volume of the oxygen at the positive pole; water, therefore, is composed in bulk of one volume of oxygen and two volumes of hydrogen; but oxygen being sixteen times as heavy as hydrogen, eight parts of oxygen by weight unite with one part of hydrogen to form water. We may justly term water an *oxide of hydrogen*.

Water exists in Nature in three forms; in the solid as ice, in the liquid as water, and in the gaseous as steam. The greater part of the water existing in Nature is undergoing a slow but constant process of distillation, condensation, and redistillation; it rises from the evaporation of the waters of the earth in the form of steam, to become clouds; these again condense and fall as rain, sleet, snow, or hail.

Rain-water is the purest form of water occurring in Nature; however, even during its fall to the surface of the earth, it acquires impurities from the air, but directly it touches the land it falls upon, it dissolves some of the materials with which it comes in contact, and becomes still more impure. Most salts are more or less soluble in water, which is the most general solvent of chemical substances in Nature; rain-water thus dissolves and combines with portions of the soluble constituents from the strata through which it percolates, and becomes spring-water or river-water, and ultimately passes into the sea, to again take part in this vast process of distillation. The solid matter in solution in water is deposited when the water is evaporated; in order to obtain pure water, it is therefore necessary to *distil* it, that is, to boil it, and collect the water produced by the condensation of the steam.

So great are the solvent properties of distilled water, that when water is distilled in glass or earthenware vessels, it dissolves small quantities of the substance of the vessel in which it is condensed; and if retorts be so arranged that distillation and redistillation from one vessel to the other may be carried on, and further, if this process is often repeated, a sediment will be found at the bottom of each vessel. The sediment formed part of the vessels in which the process was carried on, was dissolved by the water on its condensation, and was deposited when it evaporated; and the oftener the distillation is repeated, the greater is the deposit.

This fact led many of the Grecian philosophers to refer all things to water, for they conceived that solid matter *originated* even from distilled water. In fact, that all solid matter was at one time in aqueous solution.

The process of boiling spring-water, or river-water, precipitates part of the solid matter it contains, especially those salts which are held in solution by an excess of carbonic acid (if carbonates be present).

Most drinking waters[*] contain *lime* to a greater or a less extent, in some form or other, generally as carbonate, or sulphate; and those waters which contain lime to any extent should be avoided for drinking purposes. The *alkaline* salts contained in many waters do not accumulate in the system; they are, therefore, not injurious, but many of them are beneficial.

[*] London water contains from 15 to 18 grains of lime per gallon. Its use for drinking purposes tends to shorten life to an extent greater than would be generally imagined.

There are many recorded cases of longevity which may be distinctly traced to drinking large quantities of water.

The Seres, expressly called *Macrobii*, or the ancient Chinese, lived to extraordinary ages, and Lucian ascribes their longevity to their "drinking water in great abundance."

The idea which was held centuries ago, that dew* water collected from the mountains, and used as a drink, would prolong life, is a very correct one; it is a distilled water of Nature, and whether it is charged with electricity or not, is very invigorating.

Distilled water, used as a drink, is absorbed directly into the blood, the solvent properties of which it increases to an extent that it will keep salts already existing in the blood in solution, prevent their undue deposition in the various organs and structures, and favour their elimination by the different excretæ. If the same be taken in large quantities, or if it be the only liquid taken into the system, either as a drink or as a medium for the ordinary decoctions of tea, coffee, etc., it will in time tend to remove those earthy compounds which have accumulated in the system, the effects of which usually become more manifest as the age of forty or fifty years is attained.

The daily use of distilled water facilitates the removal of deleterious compounds from the body

* Dew is the condensation of the aqueous vapour by a body which has *radiated* its atomic motion of heat below the temperature of the surrounding atmosphere. Its solvent power was known to the Rosicrucians, who used morning dew as a drink.

PROLONGATION OF EXISTENCE. 181

by means of the excretæ, and therefore tends to the prolongation of existence.

The use of distilled water may be especially recommended after the age of thirty-five or forty years is attained; it will of itself prevent many diseases to which mankind is especially subject after this age; and were it generally used, gravel, stone in the bladder, and other diseases due to the formation of calculi in different parts of the system, would be much more-uncommon.

Vessels, or retorts, used for the distillation of water for drinking purposes, should be made of iron,[*] not of glass or earthenware.

Lactic acid is produced by natural or artifical fermentation from milk, or other animal matter, containing lactose, or milk-sugar. In a pure state it is a syrupy liquid, transparent, and inodorous, soluble in water, alcohol, and ether. When distilled, it decomposes, unless atmospheric air be excluded, when it may be distilled unchanged.

Milk holds in solution cheese or caseine, the solubility of which is dependent upon the presence of *alkaline phosphates*, and *free alkalies*, and not upon *earthy* salts. The neutralisation of the alkali by an acid causes the cheese to separate. Fermentation may be naturally or artifically communicated to the milk-sugar which is present in the milk, the elements of which are transposed into lactic acid, which

---

[*] A distilling apparatus made of iron may be procured of Potter and Sons, 361, Oxford Street, W.

neutralises the alkali, and causes the caseine to separate.

The caseine, or cheese-curd, contains nearly all the phosphate of lime and earthy matter, but only part of the *alkaline* phosphates of the milk; but the liquid, or *whey*, contains the remaining *alkaline phosphates, lactates*, and the *lactic acid.*

Buttermilk is milk deprived of its butter, or oily part, the milk-sugar of which has been more or less converted into lactic acid. It appears to be generally given to pigs, but formerly it was largely used as an article of human consumption, and it has many good points which recommend it as a food for invalids, and as a dietetic article for more general use.*

Lactic acid forms a definite series of salts with the alkaline and *earthy* bases, and has a great tendency to prevent the undue accumulation of earthy matter in the system. There are also many instances of extraordinary longevity, which may be traced solely to lactic acid contained in whey, or buttermilk, used as a continued article of diet, several instances of which we have given in the preceding chapter.

Amongst other solvents we have the mineral acids, sulphuric, nitric, hydrochloric, and phosphoric. With the exception of the latter (phosphoric acid), the mineral acids, in large quantities, are foreign to the system, and their continued use is injurious. The action of phosphoric acid will be entered into when we consider phosphorus.

* Koumiss is a good substitute, and at the same time more palatable.

Amongst those substances which prevent the excessive action of atmospheric oxygen or the waste of the system, we first notice *tannin*, which has the power of tanning, hardening, and rendering the albuminous gelatinous structures of the body more leather-like in character, and less liable to decay.*

Tannic and gallic acids alone are objectionable, and their continued use produces dyspepsia. Their combination with an alkali to a certain extent removes

* When we consider that for a long period the natives of almost every country have resorted to the use of vegetable infusions as tea, coffee, or chocolate, it must be from some physiological demand. In Central and South America both the Indian and the Creole indulge in chocolate. The North American Indians have their Apallachian and other teas, and in the West Indies and United States the Europeans drink their coffee. The same with France, Belgium, Turkey, Germany, and Sweden. England and Russia substitute tea; the same with China and other Asiatic countries. The followers of Mahomet drink coffee, and even in Central Africa we find the Abyssinian chaat. Wherever we travel we find some native beverage; and what is more curious, they are almost identical in chemical composition.

They all contain a volatile oil upon which their aroma is dependent; a nitrogenous compound, as *theine*, *caffeine*, and *theobromine*; and also an *astringent acid*, of which the *tannic acid* of tea is a good example.

With the addition of oxygen and water, the nitrogenous constituents yield taurine, a constituent of the bile. Theine is closely related to kreatinine, which is found in the muscular system of warm-blooded animals, so that these beverages present a remarkable resemblance to soups in their vivifying power.

The experiments of Lehmann in 1854 showed that when the infusion of three-quarters of an ounce of coffee was taken daily for fourteen days "the amount of urea and phosphoric acid excreted by the kidneys was less by one-third than when the same food was taken without the coffee." His opinion was that it retarded the waste of the tissues of the body, and such is undoubtedly the case, for we have a nitrogenous principle which helps to nourish, and at the same time an this objection, and they exist in Nature, combined with *potash*, in the walnut, acorn, etc., the action of which we have already noticed when speaking of the longevity and diet of the ancient Britons.

Potash alum, a combination of sulphate of alumina and sulphate of potash, has a similar astringent action if taken in small doses. This remark does not apply to the *ammonia* alum, which is generally used in the present day on account of its cheapness; sulphate of ammonia, which is largely produced in our gas-works, is here substituted for the sulphate of potash of the potash alum.

astringent one, which, by combining chemically with the gelatinous tissues of the body, hardens them, and prevents their waste and decay. There is therefore a philosophical reason why 100 millions of people drink coffee, 55 millions cocoa, 10 to 20 millions infusions of a similar nature, and over 500 millions tea.

In some of these beverages it is found by experience that the amount of astringent matter is sometimes too great for assimilation. Thus those persons who drink strong decoctions of tea in large quantities, suffer from a peculiar dyspepsia, owing to the tannin acting on the coats of the stomach and retarding its secretions. This has necessitated the use of a substance which would combine with it and prevent its injurious action. Milk has been found one of the best liquids for this purpose, and although the chemical principle has never been clearly explained it is very simple.

The tannin of the tea combines with the albuminoid constituents of the milk, and forms a temporarily insoluble substance, part of which is subsequently digested and assimilated by the body, without any pernicious action occurring.

The Chinese allow their tea to stand only for a few minutes, therefore only a portion of the tannin is extracted, and it can be taken without milk.

The Russian system of taking lemon-juice in tea is also a good one, because the presence of citric acid prevents the astringent action on the coats and glands of the stomach.

The majority of these infusions delay the process of digestion.

PROLONGATION OF EXISTENCE.

Fresh brewers' yeast has a great affinity for oxygen, and would undoubtedly prevent undue oxidation or waste of the tissues. Within the last few years it has been employed medicinally, with good effect, in many diseases which are characterised by excessive oxidation.

The alkalies, *potash* and *soda*, have the property of increasing the solubility of albumen and fibrin. The continued use of soda is depressing. The best preparation of the alkalies for this purpose is the liquor potassæ, in small doses of five or ten drops, largely diluted with water. It acts also as an antacid and antilithic; but its continued use renders the fluids and urine so alkaline, that deposits of earthy phosphates may possibly result from this alkalinity; but this deposit, which is chiefly noticeable in the urine, is dependent solely upon diet—or the quantity of earthy phosphates taken into the system as food, and is to a great extent preventible by the conjoined use of the vegetable acids, and entirely by phosphoric acid, as a citrate, tartrate, or phosphate. Phosphoric acid undergoes no alteration in passing through the system, and is therefore traceable to the secretions and excretions. But vegetable acids are not found in either; they are, as it were, burnt up in the system, and resolved into carbonic acid and water. This action *lowers* the temperature of the body and increases the fluidity of the blood, and this is the reason that the vegetable acids act so beneficially in many forms of fever, and not because they neutralise ammonia, which is found in excess in the blood in most fevers, and which neutralisation, did it exist, could only last for a short period.

The vegetable acids, either alone or combined with alkalies as they exist in fruits, or artificially prepared, as before stated, tend to prolong life—firstly, by decreasing the temperature of the body, therefore the waste of the system; secondly, on the combustion of the acid, the alkali being left free, the solubility of albumen and fibrine existing in both the blood and the tissues is increased, there is a lessened tendency to their deposit—to the formation of fibrinous and gelatinous accumulations in the system.*

* Some few years ago an article appeared in the *Daily Telegraph* under the heading "The Way to Live for Ever." It was a review of a treatise entitled *Makrobiotik and Eubanic: two Scientific Methods for the Prolongation and Embellishment of Human Life*, by Dr. Wilhelm Schmoele, Professor of Pathology in Germany. The following are some extracts:

"The transmutation of metals, quadrature of the circle, and perpetual motion, still remain unsolved mysteries, probably because Dr. Schmoele has not yet turned his attention to them; but the Elixir of Life stands revealed to us by his patient and laborious researches into the arcana of Nature.

"It was reserved to Dr. Schmoele to gladden the world with the disclosure that *lemon-juice* is the Elixir Vitæ . . . to eat a fixed number of lemons having relation to his or her age or sex every morning and evening.

"He confidently hopes in future ages, far remote, to supply posterity with an illustration in his own person of his theory, that '*he who will only eat lemons enough need never die.*'

"Count Weldeck died in Paris, aged 120 years, and every springtide he was in the habit of devouring horseradish soaked in lemon-juice in large quantities. 'It was not the horseradish,' says Dr. Schmoele, 'but the lemon-juice which prolonged his life for so many years.'

"Between fifty and sixty, the dose for ladies is set down at three,

PROLONGATION OF EXISTENCE.

Amongst the agents which combine the *two* actions, the only one we can recommend is *phosphorus*, because it is a substance not foreign to the system. When phosphorus is in a *free* state, owing to its great affinity for oxygen it unites with it in the system, thereby decreasing the waste, decomposition, or oxidation of the body, and forms acids which prevent the accumulation of earthy compounds, and facilitate their elimination from the system.

Phosphorus, owing to its great affinity for oxygen, does not occur free in Nature, except in the most highly organised structures of animals and a few plants; apart from these, it exists only in a state of combination always with oxygen, and with an alkaline or earthy base, generally as phosphate of lime, which is found largely in mountains in Spain and

for 'gentlemen four lemons a day. One lemon more per diem is ordained to each sex for every additional decade. So that a person would soon be busily engaged eating lemons all day, and would ere long ask himself the question, 'Is life worth living?' Lemon-juice would act as a solvent for the lime contained in horseradish or other vegetable matter, on the same principle that you can dissolve pearl and similar substances in it. This action could only exist before the substance was swallowed, for the acid would, in the system, be resolved into carbonic acid and water, leave the lime behind, or deposited, and not act as a solvent for any calcareous matter in the system. The active principle of the lemon is citric acid, which does not remove lime from the system, but its decomposition lowers the temperature of the body, therefore the waste, so that it indirectly tends to prolong life, but not to the extent imagined by Dr. Schmoele. Phosphorus, phosphoric acid, and several other substances are much more efficacious, and scientifically more correct in principle. We fear that the imbibition of large quantities of lemon-juice will not herald the approach of the period when, as Sir Walter Scott says, 'Sages shall become monarchs of the earth; and death itself retreat from their frown.'"

other parts of the world. Phosphate of lime is the principal constituent of apatite, phosphorite, coprolites, etc., and exists in most structures throughout the animal and vegetable kingdoms; and, in conjunction with other earthy compounds, plays a great part in causing their death by its accumulation.

In the animal kingdom it is taken into the system in the articles of diet derived generally from vegetables; and, in the vegetable kingdom, by imbibition or absorption from the earth.

Phosphorus was accidentally discovered by Brandt, of Hamburg, in 1669; but Scheele obtained it from bones, and examined its properties, in 1769. It is generally prepared from powdered bone-ash, or phosphate of lime, by adding to it about two-thirds of its weight of sulphuric acid and about sixteen parts of water. By this means the bone-ash is decomposed; the sulphuric acid unites with part of the lime, forming sulphate of lime, which is insoluble and precipitates, whilst the greater part of the phosphorus is left in combination with oxygen, hydrogen, and the remaining lime, forming superphosphate of lime which remains in solution. This solution is then evaporated to the consistence of a syrup, and mixed with charcoal; it is then placed in earthenware retorts, the necks of which, to prevent the admission of atmospheric oxygen, are placed under water. It is then heated to redness, when carbonic oxide is liberated, and the phosphorus distils over and falls as yellowish drops to the bottom of the water.

The phosphorus thus prepared is generally purified by redistillation, and by pressing it through leather under hot water; but the phosphorus thus purified generally contains so many impurities that it is unfit for medicinal use. The chief impurity is arsenic, but bismuth, copper, and cobalt are often found in what is known as "commercial" phosphorus. For internal use it therefore requires further purification. When phosphorus has been passed through leather, boiling in *liquor potassæ* will readily remove the arsenic, forming a *liquor arsenicalis*. It should then be mixed with vegetable charcoal, redistilled, and allowed to fall into lime-water. It should then be washed, or well agitated, in *liquor ammoniæ fortis*. What slight impurities may now be present, will readily be removed by adding a mixture composed of equal parts of charcoal and *carbonate of iron*, making this into a paste and redistilling, when irregular masses of *pure* phosphorus are obtained.

Phosphorus readily oxidises, and slight friction, or sometimes the heat of the hand, will cause its ignition. It unites with oxygen in two proportions. With oxygen and hydrogen in five.

"When phosphorus is kept for a time near its boiling-point, air being excluded, it undergoes a *true coagulation*, and, at the same time, a change in its most striking properties."—LIEBIG.

If common phosphorus be exposed to a temperature between 464° and 482° Fah., for some hours, atmospheric air being excluded, or in an atmosphere such as hydrogen or carbonic acid, which will not act chemically on it, it becomes a solid dark red and opaque substance, exactly *equal in weight* to the common phosphorus used, but differing greatly from it in properties. This is what is called *amorphous phosphorus*.

The ordinary phosphorus is easily fusible, very inflammable in contact with air, is luminous in the dark, is readily oxidised, and slowly passes in the air into a deliquescent acid; whilst the altered, red, or amorphous phosphorus is not inflammable, and does not take fire until sufficient heat is used to reconvert it into the ordinary form; it is not luminous, and it is not changed in moist air.

Bisulphuret of carbon dissolves common phosphorus in all proportions, but the altered phosphorus is insoluble in it.

Common phosphorus has distinct actions upon the animal system, and, in excess, is very poisonous; the same quantity of the altered phosphorus is inert, and has no action whatever on the body.

At a *low red heat*, the altered or amorphous phosphorus is *reconverted* into the ordinary form.

"Now, what is the *cause* of these transformations in the properties of this element? What is the mysterious part played here by heat? We can explain difference of properties in two compounds of the same composition, by a difference in the arrangement of their atoms; and this view in many cases is unquestionably correct. But how is it with phosphorus, which we must regard as an elementary body? *Is phosphorus, perhaps, really a compound?* These remarkable phenomena are as yet obviously unexplained; but they open up to us a world of new ideas."—LIEBIG.

Phosphorus *in the air* gives off white fumes, which are luminous in the dark: these fumes are due to combustion or oxidation; but phosphorus is luminous *in vacuo*, and the more complete the vacuum, the greater is the luminosity. Here oxygen plays no part—phosphorus is luminous *per se;* its luminosity, therefore, is not necessarily due to oxidation.

If albumen or white of egg be kept for a time at its boiling-point, it coagulates; *a something* (a vitality?) imperceptible, imponderable, and not necessarily chemical, has gone—it is eliminated by the heat, and the character and properties of the albumen are changed. This *something*, or a something analogous, may be given back to it either by animal digestion, or artificially by chemical means, when its former properties are restored, and it becomes again true or fluid albumen coagulable by heat.

When phosphorus is kept for some hours at its boiling-point, "it undergoes a true coagulation;" a *something** imperceptible and imponderable has gone.

---

* A similar instance is seen in the diamond, although "when heated strongly in a medium incapable of acting chemically upon it, the diamond swells up, and is converted into a black mass resembling coke," and also, when burnt in oxygen, carbonic acid alone is formed—showing it to consist of pure carbon. The diamond is not pure carbon alone, for a *something* imponderable is driven off by heat, and pure

The weight is exactly the same; but the continued heat has eliminated a *something*, and the properties of the phosphorus are changed. A higher temperature gives back this *something*, and the phosphorus again assumes its former characters. But as phosphorus on its combustion gives off electricity, we may justly infer that this *something* which is eliminated is *electricity*. Again, as phosphorus is luminous in a vacuum, totally independent of oxidation, it would be neither theoretical nor speculative to say that we need not regard phosphorus as an elementary body, but that it is really a compound, of which *light* in the abstract form and *electricity* are important constituents.

The light in this case is light *per se*—it does not originate in heat—the motion of the radiation of atoms; nor does it arise from combustion or any combination of gases. It is luminous when removed from all chemical action.

It has been shown in the present century that *light* is an originator of motion; this is instanced in the little instrument invented by Mr. Crooke, which rotates under the influence of the sun's rays, and the more intense the light, the greater the rapidity of the

carbon is left exactly the same in weight as the diamond; we have, therefore, discovered the means of eliminating this *something* from the diamond, but we have not as yet been able to replace it, or to unite carbon and this imponderable something. When this is discovered, we shall be able to make diamonds artificially: and were a man to make this end his object, we see nothing to prevent his success. Its discoverer would perhaps be struck with amazement, but he might also be amused at its simplicity.

motion. This instrument is constructed for the purpose, and instances the action of light upon *dead* matter; what, therefore, may be the influence of light upon *living* matter!

Phosphorus exists in the most highly developed organs or structures of man and animals.

"The *brain* and other nerve-centres contain a substance termed *protagon*, of which *phosphorus* forms an essential constituent. It crystallises in microscopic needles, and is very easily decomposed. Amongst the *products* of decomposition of protagon are glycerine, *phosphoric acid*, and several fatty acids, and an ammonium base called *neurine*."—ROSCOE.

Now, certain proportions of phosphorus exist in the brain in a free or unoxidised form, and within the last few years we see it stated that the protagon of the brain and nervous system contains its phosphorus as a hypophosphite. This error may easily be accounted for from the fact that protagon readily decomposes, and the phosphorus combining with oxygen, would be found as a hypophosphite, or even as a phosphate or as phosphoric acid, if the brain were not in a fresh state. However, difference of opinion is not needed on this point, as a very simple experiment will decide the question.

If we take a *fresh* brain (either human or animal), and immerse it in either absolute alcohol, sulphuric ether, or olive oil, we obtain a *luminous* solution of phosphorus; a phosphate is not luminous, a hypophosphite is not luminous, *free* phosphorus is luminous. The brain, therefore, contains free or unoxidised phosphorus.

We naturally inquire for what purpose phosphorus exists in this form, in the largest quantity, in structures of the highest organisation — as, for instance, the brain, which, as an established physiological fact, presides over every thought and action of our material bodies.

The first *cause* of thought is not organic, it has a higher origin, the nature of which we are as yet unacquainted with; and as Hufeland, a philosophic physician, said a century ago, "The first *cause* of *thought* is spiritual; but the *business of thinking* itself, as carried on in this mortal machine, is *organic*."

Now, the brain contains cells, some larger than others, and variously shaped. The brain also contains fibres, some of which are tubular, and have a covering membrane, and some of which have not, called respectively *tubular* and *gelatinous* fibres. Some of these fibres are joined to and issue from the cells; this is undoubtedly the case with some of the *caudate* or larger cells, which have tail-like processes, some of which "become continuous, with an ordinary nerve fibre." This is not always the case, nor is it necessary to have direct continuity. Contact is all we require; and most, if not all, the fibres of the brain are in *contact* with cells. Here in the brain, spinal marrow, and nerves, we see a most perfect *telegraphic* apparatus—Nature's design, and which is distributed

PROLONGATION OF EXISTENCE.

by means of the nerves and their subdivisions—arborescent ramifications to every part of the body, and which we may compare to a set of *telegraph wires*.

During thought, mental exertion, worry, remorse, or hard study, *phosphates* are largely increased in the excretæ; and as the brain is the centre of these thoughts and ideas, we may justly infer that this increase of phosphates is due to oxidation or loss of phosphorus from the brain—that the *first* effect of thought is to cause oxidation of phosphorus during the "*business of thinking* itself."

Now, it is a chemico-physiological fact that the brain contains phosphorus.

It is a chemical fact that on the oxidation or burning up of phosphorus in the atmosphere an electric charge is given off.

It is a demonstrable fact that on passing a current of electricity along the course of one or more nerves of an animal body, spasmodic actions, muscular contractions, are the result.

It is, therefore, clear that phosphorus plays a more important action in the animal economy than has heretofore been supposed; and that thought, the mind itself, many nervous actions with which the mind has no connection, and volition and common sensation, are intimately connected with the presence of phosphorus in the cerebro-spinal axis.

As an instance of this we may ask: What is *motion* caused by will? A man puts forth his hand to reach a certain object. Phosphorus is oxidised in the brain in cells, which either communicate or are in contact with nerve fibres, and the electric* current caused by the oxidation of phosphorus in the brain passes down these fibres (on exactly the same principle as the telegraph wire) to the arm or hand, contractions of muscles in the limb result—the action he willed is completed.

"Every thought, every sensation, is accompanied by a change in the composition of the substance of the brain."—LIEBIG.

"According to careful estimates, three hours of hard study wear out the body more than a whole day of hard physical exertion. 'Without phosphorus, no thought,' is a German saying; and the consumption of that essential ingredient of the brain increases in proportion to the amount of labour which this organ is required to perform. The wear and tear of the brain are easily measured by careful examination of the salts of the liquid excretions."—*Boston Journal of Chemistry*.

* In the study of an eminent philosopher, named De Luc, a suspended ball was kept in regular pulsation for years by means of successive accumulations of electricity from a dry pile, the discharges being carried off by the ball. Phosphorus must of necessity be gradually oxidised in the cerebro-spinal axis, even in sleep; electricity must develop, and when it has reached a certain tension, must be discharged along the nerves which supply the heart, and thus cause its pulsation, and the resulting circulation of the blood. A similar conclusion was arrived at by Sir John Herschel, also by Dr. Arnott; but neither of them showed a *source* of the required electrical power.

The importance of the brain is again verified by the fact that although it only weighs, on an average, one-fortieth of the weight of the body, one-fifth of the blood goes to supply this organ. Now does the brain, as is generally believed, derive its supply of phosphorus from earthy or alkaline phosphates taken into the system in the articles of diet? Is there any action existing in the body which has the power to de-oxidise phosphates and extract free phosphorus?

"The mean temperature of man is 98° 6';" and the only means we have at present of artificially preparing phosphorus from phosphates is by detaching the oxygen by charcoal at a *red heat*, a temperature which could not exist in any living organism; nor is there any electric action in the body of sufficient force for this purpose.

"*Light* separates the moisture in plants into its constituent hydrogen and oxygen, and it disengages the oxygen from the carbonic acid, so as to deposit the carbon in union with hydrogen—as gum, resin, and oil, which forms their ligneous parts. Consolidation and vigour *depend on light*."

"The retention of oxygen, for want of *light*, renders plants white.... Solar light is the agent by which the carbonic acid in gas is decomposed."

"The life of every created being is the more perfect the more it enjoys the influence of *light*. Let a plant or an animal be deprived of light, notwithstanding every nourishment, care, and cultivation, it will first lose its colour, then its strength, and at last entirely decay. Even man who passes his life in darkness becomes pale, relaxed, and heavy, and at length loses the whole *energy of life;* as is proved by the many melancholy instances of persons shut up in gloomy dungeons."

In darkness there is no expansion of organised life except at the expense of putrefaction and decomposition, resulting only in the production of vegetation of the most imperfect kind; apart from this, no form of life is generated of a higher order—nothing feels, nothing breathes.

"The phosphoric light seen in the ocean is caused by innumerable quantities of *phosphoric* insects (*noctiluca miliaris*), and is sometimes so intense as to make the waves appear like red-hot balls."

"Owen describes cylindrical flexible mollusca, in the sea near Benguela, a foot long, and two inches in diameter, which, agitated, become *vividly luminous.*"

Fire-flies are very common in Mexico and South America, and a similar species is found in Africa; they "shine by so strong a *phosphoric* light that a person may read by the light of three of them."

Some of these insects have three luminous patches, one on each side of the head, and one on the under part of the body. The light continues *for some time* after the fly is dead. The light of the *glow-worm* is too well known to need description. The light is only emitted when they are in motion, and it arises from the last two rings of the abdomen. "Their remains are *phosphorescent*."

"*Luminosity* has been noticed chiefly in fungi. A species of argaric, in Western Australia, is said to afford a phosphorescent light of sufficient intensity to read by. Decaying wood, called *touchwood*, caused by the mycelium of fungi, is often phosphorescent; and in Brazil certain mushrooms give out a light like that of fire-flies."

The snail, millepedes, and other insects are distinctly luminous in the dark, as are the mackerel, herring, and many other fish.

Von Humboldt, speaking of the *medusæ* found in sea-water, says: "They observed, after it became dark, that none of the three species of medusæ which they had collected emitted light unless they were slightly shaken. When a very irritable individual is placed on a tin plate, and the latter is struck with a piece of metal, the vibrations of the tin are sufficient to make the animal shine. Sometimes, on galvanising medusæ, the phosphorescence appears at the moment when the chain closes, although the exciters are not in direct contact with the body of the subject. The *fingers, after touching it, remain luminous* for two or three minutes. Wood, on being *rubbed* with a medusa, *becomes luminous*, and after the phosphorescence has ceased it may be *rekindled by passing the dry hand over it*." Again, "On their return to the latter of these (Gaurabo), the travellers were much struck by the prodigious number of *phosphorescent* insects which illuminated the grass and foliage. These insects (*elater noctilucus*) are occasionally used for a lamp, being placed in a calabash perforated with holes; and a young woman at Trinidad informed them that, during a long passage from the mainland, she always had recourse to this *light* when she gave her child the breast at night, the captain not allowing any other on board, for fear of pirates."

We have ourselves seen the grass, shrubs, and underwood of forests in Africa brightly illuminated and glittering with *luminous* insects; and the waves of the ocean brilliant with vivid fire from the light emitted by species of medusæ; and, where we have been enabled to procure specimens, we found that in most of them the light was phosphorescent; in many cases, the fingers remained luminous after touching them, and from many we were enabled to obtain luminous solutions of phosphorus in an oxidisable form.

Now do these numerous *luminous* beings of animated nature, both vegetable and animal, obtain their phosphorus from phosphates?

As it is our desire to avoid theory or speculation until we have sufficient evidence to say positively "yes" or "no," we will leave the subject of the *source* of the *phosphorus* existing in the brain and other structures of man, by asking the following questions:

1. Does man "by a chemical decomposition, the nature of which it is not easy to explain," extract the phosphorus existing in his system from phosphates contained in the articles of his diet?

2. Does he obtain it partly from phosphates, and partly from elsewhere?

3. Does he derive it solely from *another* source?

Whatever the *source* of the phosphorus of the brain may be, it is clear that it must first exist in the blood, and be carried by it to the brain, which we may therefore compare to a *gland*, one purpose of which is for the secretion or absorption of phosphorus from the blood—to collect it and fix it in its own substance, for the purpose of taking part in some of the most important functions and manifestations of the vital phenomena — both perceptible and imperceptible—incidental to, and essentially part of, that as yet incomprehensible and indefinable condition which we term *Life:* the elements or the materials of which it is built we may eventually become thoroughly acquainted with, but the plan will remain obscure—the design is known to the Architect alone.

Direct experiment, and many records on the chemical pathology of the brain, show that although phosphates by their gradual deposition often increase in the brain, the quantity of oxidisable phosphorus *decreases* in " old age."

The foregoing few remarks on phosphorus we have made to show the great importance of this substance in the animal economy—to briefly demonstrate the interesting and instructive properties and manifest influence which it bears towards many of the observed and comprehensible phenomena of organic life, in the hope that many of these phenomena may not long remain questions or problems for futurity to solve; and further to verify the statement which we made in our first chapter, that "this great vital principle, which is centred in the cerebro-spinal axis, gradually wanes, because the brain and nerves by degrees lose their supply of blood, their powers of selection and imbibition, and are deprived of their ordained nourishment, by means of this gradual process of induration and ossification."

We do not state that phosphorus is itself a vital principle, but that it plays an important part in the phenomena of organic life; and as the brain must of necessity derive its supply of phosphorus from the blood, which circulates in vessels which, as we have already shown, gradually indurate, ossify, and become lessened in calibre as age advances, so must the brain and nerves gradually lose their powers of selection and imbibition, and be deprived of their ordained nourishment—and so does the quantity of oxidisable phosphorus in the brain decrease in "old age." Hence the gradual impairment of the functions of the brain and nerves, and the numerous actions dependent, directly or indirectly, upon these delicate and exquisitely formed organs.

The reason that phosphorus, which, as Majendie

says, "would seem to have effected almost resurrections," has been so little regarded, is entirely owing to the want of a reliable preparation.

In the present day it is used in the form of "pills," combined with balsam of tolu, yellow wax, and similar vehicles; it is also used dissolved in sulphuric ether, chloroform, rectified alcohol, etc.; and it is also given internally in solution in almond, olive, and cod-liver oils.

If water is added to the ethereal or alcoholic solutions, the phosphorus precipitates. In the form of pills it is insoluble in water; also insoluble in the blood, and little, if any, of the phosphorus in these preparations is really absorbed into, and assimilated by, the system. Again, owing to the inflammability of phosphorus in the solid form, it may produce inflammation and even ulceration of the stomach and bowels; we may therefore unhesitatingly say, that any form of phosphorus where *solid particles* are either present or are produced by the addition of water, is, to say the least, unreliable and uncertain in its action, and may be dangerous in its use. Even in solution in oil, we have on one occasion seen sufficient irritation produced, to result in a disease analogous in appearance and characters to erysipelas.*

It is therefore only just and correct to state that

---

* This may be due to the particles of oil holding phosphorus in solution, and incapable of further subdivision, being arrested in the capillaries supplying the skin.

the preparations of phosphorus generally used are not satisfactory in their results.

Thick syrup, mucilage, and several similar compounds have the property of retaining free phosphorus—not in mechanical, but in aqueous solution—if transmitted to them by means of a proper medium or volatile solvent. As an instance, if we dissolve in sulphuric ether as much phosphorus as the ether will take up, and add, we will say, from thirty to sixty drops of this solution to a pint of thick syrup, shake them together, allow the ether to evaporate, and decant the greater portion of the syrup, leaving a small quantity at the bottom of the vessel, which retains what solid particles of phosphorus may have precipitated, the upper or decanted part is perfectly clear and transparent, and will be found to contain in aqueous—not in mechanical—solution sufficient phosphorus, even in doses of one or two drachms, to distinctly influence and increase the amount of phosphates in the liquid excretions.

By using glycerine instead of the syrup, we may obtain even a stronger preparation than the above. Here we have two preparations of phosphorus in aqueous solution, and although they contain but a small proportion, it is in a form which cannot precipitate, and which may be readily absorbed into the system. Small doses only are required, for the whole is assimilated, whereas in most of the preparations in which a thirty-sixth or even a twentieth part of a grain per dose are given, only a fraction serves its desired use, and the remaining portion is often passed out of the system unchanged.

In the present age of rapidity and despatch, phosphorus is often a deficient constituent of the brain and nerves. It is often wasted in the turmoil of business, in anxious moments pending loss or success, in grief and sadness, and the acute trials arising from family and other bereavements; in the mental applications and exertions of the scholar, to whatever section of science he may be attached; in even the excessive indulgences and libations of the inebriate, who delights in the stimulant and unconsciously in the solvent properties of alcohol—which in excess dissolves and removes phosphorus from his brain—hence the tremor and other symptoms dependent upon a deficiency of nerve power.

To demonstrate the action of phosphorus upon the system, after its absorption into the blood, we may divide it into two portions. One part is carried by the circulation to the brain, which assimilates and fixes it in its own substance; thus serving to take part in—even to increase—many of the mental and nervous phenomena of organic life. The other part is carried by the general circulation to every structure and organ of the body. During its passage it fixes and combines with oxygen existing in the blood, and becomes hypophosphorus, afterwards phosphoric acid.

Phosphorus therefore combines with oxygen existing in the blood, and by this means *prevents excessive oxidation* or waste of the system; again, when on its union with oxygen it becomes phosphoric acid, it combines with the alkaline and *earthy* bases existing in the blood, forming neutral salts; and further, as the amount of phosphoric acid increases, part of the insoluble earthy compounds (which have been gradually deposited) become superphosphates, which are soluble—which circulate again in the blood, and part of which are *removed from the system* in the liquid excretions—thus *preventing the accumulation of earthy compounds* in the system, and even *removing those which have* been already *deposited*.

Phosphorus, therefore, by its great affinity for oxygen, prevents the undue accumulation of fibrinous and gelatinous substances in the system, and on its becoming phosphoric acid, removes the earthy matter which has gradually accumulated—which we have termed "ossification"—which is the chief *cause* of "old age," and "natural death;" thereby, in the full sense of the term, *prolonging life for a lenghened period!*

Hypophosphites have a similar action; they fix oxygen from the blood, and *become phosphates*, thus preventing undue waste of the system. This is the reason—and the only one—that the hypophosphites act so beneficially in consumption.* The *alkaline*

---

* As two of perhaps the latest views on consumption, independent of bacilli, it is stated that consumption is due to a *lack of oxidisable phosphorus* in the system; again, that it is caused by *mineral inanition*.

Now both these are *characteristics* of the disease. Atmospheric hypophosphites only are of service for the purpose now under consideration.

Phosphoric acid possesses but the one action, that of preventing undue accumulation, and of removing earthy compounds from the system, which action we have already considered. Therefore in the agents best adapted to prolong life for a *lengthened period*, we notice chiefly distilled water used daily as a drink; unoxodised phosphorus, in syrup, glycerine, etc., in doses of one or two drachms, according to the strength of the solution; the *alkaline* hypophosphites, and the dilute phosphoric acid (corresponding to ten per cent. by weight of the anhydrous acid) in doses of from ten to twenty drops, well diluted with water. These preparations may be taken two or three times daily (according to the *degree* of ossification), as an article of *diet*, and not as a *medicine*.

It would naturally be asked that, if life were prolonged by means of the diet and the agents herein mentioned, what state of body would be the concomitant of such existence?

To this we answer, that the *cause* being to a great extent *suspended*, the effect could not follow so quickly and prematurely as it otherwise would.

---

oxygen oxidises phosphorus excessively in consumption, there is therefore a lack of oxidisable phosphorus in the body. This again gives rise to an excess of phosphoric acid, which removes alkaline and earthy salts from the system; we have therefore so-called "defective mineral nutrition." But neither of these are *causes*, they are but the results— *effects*—of a distinct and demonstrable cause, as is also the formation of tubercle.—*Vide* "Consumption, a Re-investigation of its Cause," by the Author.

For the many organs and structures could not so readily harden and ossify. The numerous characteristics of "old age" could not exist to the same extent; *and a state of mental and bodily juvenescence would be maintained for a lengthened period.*

CHAPTER VII.

CONCLUSION.

SCIENCE dictates, and even the most casual observer, who — for purpose or principle — attempts to comprehend the truths and phenomena of universal Nature, unhesitatingly admits, that "every *phenomenon* has its *reason*, every *effect* its *cause*." This is a fact established and indisputable; but how often are the *laws of life* and *of death* doomed to be overlooked by the deluded, and even removed from their legitimate situation, which they of necessity embrace in forming volumes in the library of the academy of Nature! For the sake of method, we classify and arrange under many heads, which are but servitors to avoid a chaos of observations, descriptions, and deductions; the confusions thus avoided obviously present themselves, but one branch of science is dependent upon another—each forms a part, all united a whole — for Nature is one. To recognise one and ignore another portion or an entirety—each part of which is dependent upon unity —is to break a rule which remains unbroken. To say that everything dies simply because it has lived —that the age of man is *fixed* irrespective of reason or cause—is not only presumption, but confessedly a want of conception, a disbelief in what is and therefore must be, and an assault on the fixed and immutable laws of natural phenomena.

When we reflect or meditate on the progress of civilized man, we notice wonders and improvements in his surroundings, for his welfare and comfort; we discover a spirit of inquiry amongst men, a silent march of thought—a steady progress, impelled forward by an eternal law—Nature's law—experience. This law we may compare to a circle; the beginning we know not, the end we know not. This circle enlarges, expands—where is the limit? Opposition, reproach, threats, and violence can only be a temporary check; they cannot control, abate, or arrest the progress of inquiry, the keenness of research, the results of experience. But amongst the varied and expanding objects of research, is not that inquiry which appertains to the preservation of life the most important of all to humanity?

What is man without health, even if endowed with riches? Take away the latter and their accompanying luxuries—only give him health; this accomplished, the first desire is a return of the riches. But with both a word remains which we hate to utter, a thought we dread to contemplate, a thing which gives sorrow pain and grief. That word, that thought, that thing is *Death*. Even in cases where life appears a burden, how tenaciously do men cling to it! How the spirit recoils from a struggle with Death! How fondly it retains its grasp of life! Man's great desire is for

CONCLUSION.

health and long life on earth; to this there are but some few exceptions—the result of incidental impressions. "Man clings to the world as his home, and would fain live here for ever."

"And can we see the newly-turned earth of so many graves, hear the almost hourly-sounding knell that announces the departure of another soul from its bodily fabric, meet our associates clad in the garb of woe, hear of death after death among those whom we knew—perhaps respected, perhaps loved—without pausing to consider if we may not seek and haply find *more than the mere causes*, find the *means of checking* the premature dissolution that so painfully excites the deepest and most hidden sympathies of our nature?"

"*The prolongation of the life* of the people must become an essential part of family, municipal, and national policy. Although it is right and glorious to incur risks and to sacrifice life for public objects, it has always been felt that length of days is the measure, and that the completion by the people of the full term of natural existence is the groundwork, of their felicity. For untimely death is a great evil. What is so bitter as the premature death of a wife, a child, a father? What dashes to the earth so many hopes, breaks so many auspicious enterprises, as the unnatural death? The poets, as faithful interpreters of our aspirations, have always sung, that *in the happier ages of the world this source of tears shall be dried up.*"—REGISTRAR-GENERAL OF ENGLAND.

In the present day, when we are so accustomed to wonders that they no longer excite our wonder; when we send our thoughts almost round the world with the velocity of lightning; when we hear voices miles away by the agency of the telephone; the tick of a watch—even the tramp of a fly—by the microphone; when we transcribe the vibrations of sound with the precision of a mathematician; when we freeze water into ice in white hot crucibles; when we cast copper into statues without the aid of heat; when it is possible to illuminate cities without gas—with lamps devoid of flame or fire; when some of the most precious minerals are produced from their elements; when we believe that to-morrow even the diamond may be artificially produced; with all these wonders recently brought to light for the benefit of mankind, is man *himself* to be debarred from that social progress which is daily manifested? Are the achievements of science of no avail in benefiting his degenerated existence? Will not our daily-increasing knowledge of nature and the behaviour of her elements eventually tend to this end? In reference to which Liebig asks: "Is that knowledge not the *philosopher's stone*, which promises to disclose to us the laws of life, and which *must finally yield to us the means of curing diseases and of prolonging life?*"

The fields of research become richer and wider with every new discovery, which is often as precious, if not more useful than gold—actually a transmutation for the benefit and comfort of man. But as yet

CONCLUSION. 213

he has *himself* been little benefited by science, which must of necessity ultimately dictate a *means* of curing diseases and of prolonging life. Is it even just, in the present day of so-called wisdom, to ridicule the alchemists of old, who diligently laboured and searched for a "virgin earth"—a mysterious substance which would "change the baser metals to gold, and be a means of curing diseases, of restoring youth to the exhausted frame of age, and of prolonging life indefinitely"? Such a view would be utterly unjust. For the present science of chemistry owes its position, its existence—perhaps its origin—to the untiring observations and researches of the alchemists, which were instilled into them in their laborious searches for the "philosopher's stone." All they sought for exists, and may ultimately be found in the illimitable science of chemistry.

Oxygen it is, that by combining with the substance of fuel during combustion causes the consumption of that fuel. Oxygen it is, that by combining in a similar manner with the substance of the human body, chiefly during respiration, causes the waste of the system and the necessity for food. Oxygen it is, that corrodes and eats away the solid masonry of palaces, castles, mansions, and churches, and eventually crumbles them to dust. Iron bridges, marble monuments, massive structures—of whatever architecture or material—must eventually succumb to this all-destroying agent.

The Roman proverb runs, "*Tempus edax rerum,*"

Time, the consumer of all things. But Time would be of no avail without oxygen, which is really the "*edax rerum.*"

Time is also credited with the changes which take place in the human body between youth and old age; but oxygen it is which, by wasting man's tissues, necessitates his supplying himself with food, which food contains earthy and obstructive matter, which matter by accumulating in the numerous organs and structures, increases his density and rigidity, and by hardening the same produces the various characteristics, both in appearance and texture, of old age, and by stiffening his joints, that decrepitude and inactivity which, in conjunction with the induration and ossification of the numerous organs, causes the human machine gradually to move slower and slower, and ultimately to stop, and die a "natural death."

Thus it is seen that oxygen, though necessary to support life, is the primary cause, by necessitating food, of those changes which are only so many steps from the cradle to the grave. The paradox therefore exists, that even while we breathe the breath of life we also inhale the "*edax rerum,*" which only requires *Time* to bring about our destruction.

We may therefore say that *oxygen* is but the *primary cause*, because it necessitates food; and that the *earthy* and obstructive *matter* contained in that food is the immediate and *actual cause*, inasmuch as it gradually gives rise to rigidity, ossification, and death.

As a jet kept free from clogging and obstructive matter, and supplied with pure gas, will continue to burn, independent of time, "so the human body, supplied with food free from earthy and obstructive matter, will retain the flame of life."*

The beneficial effects of fruit as an article of diet, both in health and disease, cannot be overrated. In health, the apple, the pear, the grape, the strawberry, the gooseberry, the tomato,† the fig, the date, wall-fruits, the melon, and numerous others, present such a field for choice that the most capricious appetite need never be disappointed. The supply of fruit in the United Kingdom is not great, but considerable quantities of both fresh and preserved fruits are imported from all parts of the world, and are rapidly becoming popular amongst all classes; and it is to be hoped that our fellow-countrymen will gradually become more alive to the benefits to be derived from a more general and frequent use of fruits as an article of daily food.

* *Patriarchal Longevity.*
† A few years ago a writer stated that the tomato was a cause of cancer. His argument was based upon the idea that cancer was on the increase, and so was the consumption of tomatoes. As late surgeon to one of the Cancer Hospitals allows us to emphatically say that the argument and statement are equally fallacious. The tomato is one of the best articles of diet as a preventative against cancer. As a fungus grows at the expense of nitrogen, so do malignant growths on highly nitrogenous foods. The diet should contain as little nitrogen as possible. Fruits, sago, etc., are the best. When meat is given it should be *boiled*, and the *liquid* broth, soup, or beef-tea *thrown away*. It contains the irritating constituents of flesh, which encourage the growth of cancer. Tea drunkards who consume tannin in large quantities, on the one hand, and the inhabitants of certain regions, for instance, W. Africa, for dietetic reasons, seldom suffer from this disease. The chemistry of the formation of cancer points, as a remedial agent, to the salts of aluminium.

"It is surely as worth finding out what is best to feed an Englishman on as what he shall learn or believe. Yet, for the most part, we stoke the human steam engine with ashes in utter carelessness or ignorance of the waste of vital force that results. What is the staff of life? We have fed long enough on the fruit of the *Tree of Knowledge of good and evil.* It may be that, if only we could set to work like rational men, we might become as gods—free from the taint of corruption engendered by the utilization of dead and effete matter, and in time rivalling the records of the longevity of the patriarchs."—*Weekly Times and Echo.*

"When pain and anguish wring the brow," in slight and temporary indispositions, or during prolonged febrile diseases, what is more refreshing and beneficial than the juice of the luscious orange? Indeed, in many parts of the world, especially in tropical regions, the juice of the orange, taken in large quantities, has been found to be a specific for many descriptions of fever; it is, in fact, Nature's remedy, and an unsurpassed one. "The orange cure," "The grape cure," and "The strawberry cure," are chemically correct.

Cereal and farinaceous foods form the basis of the diet of so-called "vegetarians," who are not guided by any *direct* principle, except that they believe it is wrong to eat animal food. For this reason vegetarians enjoy no better health, and live no longer, than those around them. Our remarks, therefore, apply to fruits as distinct from vegetables.

We have shown a means of partially arresting the never-ceasing action of atmospheric oxygen; less food, therefore, would be necessary to support life. We have also demonstrated a means of supplying a substance which gradually becomes deficient as age advances, which deficiency is only due to the immediate and *actual* cause of old age—the accumulation of earthy matter in the system, which may also be prevented, and even removed, when already deposited. All these actions are combined in the one substance —*free phosphorus*.*

The earthy matter may be also removed by hypophosphorus acid, by phosphoric acid, and by the daily use of *distilled* water as a drink. By these means we can therefore prolong life, in the full sense of the term, for a *lengthened* period.

It has been said that "men are more often governed by words and phrases than by facts and realities;"† this is not always the case, but did a man require visible proof that another of the same age could prolong his life even to a hundred years, by the means *herein mentioned*, that sceptic would have to devise another means of prolonging his own life to enable him to see the completion of that term of years by the other.

Of all our divisions of science, perhaps the most important of all to humanity is medicine, and as one branch of science is dependent upon another, so is medicine dependent upon physiological chemistry,

---

* A preparation of syrup of phosphorus may be obtained from Pretty and Co., 1, Great Marlborough Street, London, W.

† LORD BEACONSFIELD.

and has to patiently await its advance. Medicine, as yet far from complete, is a collection of the labours of ages, and has for its own particular purpose a view to the good of mankind.

In our numerous searches for a definition of the treatment of disease, we find none so simple, clear, and may be correct, as that given seventeen hundred years ago by Galen, a physician of Pergamus, which is to supply that which is deficient by communication, and to remove that which is in excess by means of a remedy which tends to abstract it. This is a perfect definition for the removal of disease, and for the restoration of health; and when physiological chemistry is sufficiently advanced to tell us undoubtedly which elements are deficient, and which are in excess, and when we are further able to supply or remove them, then will medicine be perfect—then will it take its place as the first, foremost, and most indispensable science—the most important of all to humanity.

In relation to the bodily state of "old age," and the possibility of delaying such a state of the system, Galen's definition has been irresistibly forced upon us. For we find in old age that earthy and other solid matter is in excess, and that phosphorus is to a certain extent deficient. The remedy is to remove that which is in excess, and to restore that which is deficient.

In an oration delivered before the Medical Society of London, Sir B. W. Richardson said: "I think I am not far wrong in making the general confession, that out of all our collection of details, gathered from time immemorial, we have never as yet eliminated so much as one great and fundamental law relating to diseases as a whole."

This deficiency in the first place arises to a great extent from a general acceptance of hypotheses as explanations of phenomena. What is "discovered" to-day is so likely to be contradicted to-morrow, "for the truth lies in the statement that in medicine *experiment*, as a rule, is turned into *hypothesis*, and not into *fact*." This is the great cause of its comparatively slow progress, and wherever hypothesis is erroneous, more patience and a longer period are required to prove it to be so, than the time occupied in its construction. In the second place, this deficiency arises from the tardy development of physiological chemistry. Let us, however, not decry medicine for these reasons; let us rather strive to advance it. For, as Sir Thomas Watson so justly observes: "The profession of medicine, having for its end the common good of mankind, knows nothing of national enmities, of political strife, of sectarian divisions. Disease and pain the sole conditions of its ministry, it is disquieted by no misgivings concerning the justice or honour of its client's cause, but dispenses its peculiar benefits without stint or scruple, to men of every country and party and rank and religion, and to men of no religion at all."

In considering exclusively the subject before us, does not the action of atmospheric oxygen upon the system—especially when excessive—and also the gradual accumulation of earthy and other solid matter in the body, with its numerous and abstruse divergencies, open out to us a world of new ideas in regard to the fundamental causes of many diseases?

In conclusion, we may say, that, although the desire for long life exists as a natural, prevalent, and deeply-rooted love, there are, through continued trial and disappointment, many exceptions : in fact, the present subject is not acceptable to all. Our remarks are therefore confined to those who believe that, "In this world there is, or might be, more sunshine than rain, more joy than sorrow, more love than hate, more smiles than tears. The good heart, the tender feeling, and the pleasant disposition make smiles, love, and sunshine everywhere."

In the pages of Nature are distinctly and legibly written—to those who will refer but with patience—the laws of life and the laws of death ; and in clear, unmistakable characters the reason—the cause—of the *ultimate* death of every animate being. There are abundant materials for investigation and research ; the cause of "old age" in man is demonstrated, and a means of *checking* it has herein been clearly explained ; and it would not be contrary to the dictates of our nature to hope that *science* may be incited into an inquiry for more general perfection, which may be the means of *actually conquering it:*

> "By showing conclusively and clearly,
> That Death is a stupid blunder merely,
> And not a necessity of our lives."
>
> LONGFELLOW.

APPENDIX.

OWING to the general objection to Biblical quotations being given as part of a scientific subject, we *append* the following Canonical and Apocryphal extracts, not for the purpose of proving, or necessarily to verify, but to show their coincidence with what we have demonstrated to be possible on scientific grounds :

"God created man *to be immortal*, and made him to be an image of His own eternity."

"And the Lord God commanded the man, saying, Of every tree of the garden thou *mayest* freely eat;* but of the tree of the knowledge of good and evil, thou shalt not eat of it; for in the day that thou eatest thereof *thou shalt surely die.*"

"And the woman said unto the serpent, We may eat of the *fruit of the trees* of the garden; but of the tree which is in the midst of the garden, God hath said, Ye shall not eat of it, neither shall ye touch it, *lest ye die.*"

"And unto Adam He said, Because thou hast hearkened unto the voice of thy wife, and hast eaten of the tree, of which I commanded thee, saying, Thou shalt *not* eat of it; cursed is the *ground* for thy sake; in sorrow shalt thou *eat of it* all the days of thy life."

* Hebrew : "*Eating, thou shalt eat.*"

"And the Lord God said, Behold the man is become as one of Us, to know good and evil; and now, LEST *he* put forth his hand, and *take also of the tree of life*, and eat, and LIVE FOR EVER: therefore the Lord God sent him forth from the Garden of Eden, to till the ground from whence he was taken."

"For God made not death: *neither hath He pleasure* in the destruction of the living."

"For He created all things that they might have their being: and the generations of the world *were* healthful: and there is no poison of destruction in them, nor the *kingdom of death* upon the earth."

"But ungodly men with their works and words called it to them."

"And (our fathers) received the *laws of life*, which they kept not."

"Know this therefore, that they which are left behind are more blessed than they that be dead."

"If therefore thou shalt destroy him, which with so great labour was fashioned, it is an easy thing to be ordained by Thy commandment, that the thing which was made might be *preserved*."

"Oh, thou Adam! what hast thou done? for though it was thou that sinned, thou art not fallen alone, but we that come of thee."

"For what profit is it unto us if there be promised an immortal time, whereas we have done the works that bring death?"

"For they shall also pray unto the Lord, that He would prosper that which they give for ease, and *remedy to prolong life*."

APPENDIX. 223

"Behold I show you a mystery; *we shall not all sleep,* but we shall all be changed . . . . then shall be brought to pass the saying that is written, Death is swallowed up in victory."

"The face of the covering cast over all people, and the veil that is spread over all nations shall be destroyed, and *death swallowed up in victory.*"

"I have no pleasure in the death of him that dieth, saith the Lord God, wherefore *turn yourselves and live ye.*"

"Fools die for want of wisdom."

Members of many religious denominations believe that there will be a day when "they shall sit every man under his *vine* and under his *fig-tree*, and none shall make them afraid."

"In that day, saith the Lord of Hosts, shall ye call every man his neighbour under the *vine* and under the *fig-tree.*"

"And they shall beat their swords into ploughshares and their spears into *pruning-hooks.*"

"And they shall plant *vineyards*, and *eat the fruit of them.*"

"There shall be no more thence an infant of days, nor an old man that hath not filled his days: for the *child* shall die an *hundred* years old."

"Behold the days come, saith the Lord, that the ploughman shall *overtake* the reaper, and *the treader of grapes him that soweth seed* . . . . and they shall plant *vineyards*, and drink the wine thereof; they shall also *make gardens and eat the fruit of them.*"

"And there shall be no more death; neither sorrow, nor crying, neither shall there be any more pain."

"The last enemy that shall be destroyed is death."

That which is true is true absolutely; materially and spiritually. It cannot therefore be claimed that this language of Scripture has exclusively a spiritual reference. Whatever the objections to these quotations may be (if any), we may observe that many are led away into atheistic and materialistic views, against their own will, contrary to the very yearnings of their inner nature, by the dictates of science; they are pulled forcibly away, they are dragged by a chain composed of links, each one of which is a theory of the day, and which we may again compare to the metals. Of these links some few are golden, true, lasting and eternal; others are but as the baser metals—oxidisable, destructible. Those which are erroneous must corrode and decay—be destroyed by the advances of investigation; they must become, as it were, but as oxides of the earths, trampled upon, unnoticed, forgotten, and eventually wrapt in the cloak of oblivion.

GLOSSARY

A

Acid	A substance capable of uniting with alkalis.
Adipose	Fatty.
Adolescence	The period between puberty and maturity.
Afferent or Peripheral lacteals.	Those near the surface.
Albumenous	Containing albumen, a substance similar to white of egg.
Alimentary Canal	The tube leading from mouth to anus, through which food passes.
Amaurosis	Blindness.
Amorphous	Formless, irregular.
Amblyopia	Indistinct vision.
Anatomy	The knowledge of the structure of the body learnt by dissection.
Antiseptic	Opposed to putrefaction.
Aorta	The largest artery in the body, rising direct from the heart.
Aponeurosis	Tendon-like fibrous tissue.
Aqueous	Like water.
Arachnoid	A membrane of the brain.
Arcus senilis	An opaque circle round the cornea, observed chiefly in old people.
Arterial system	The vessels or tubes that are concerned in the circulation of arterial blood.
Artery	A tube which conveys purified or bright red blood from the heart to the capillaries.
Atheroma	Fatty degeneration of a blood vessel.
Atrophy	Wasting.

B

Bacillus	A small vegetable organism, instrumental in causing decomposition and many diseases.
Bile	A fluid secreted by the liver, playing an important part in intestinal digestion.

Bios	. .	The Greek for life.
Blastema	. .	Rudimental tissue element; protoplasm.
Bone	. .	Compact tissue forming the skeleton.

C

Caffeine	. .	The alkaloid of coffee.
Caudate	. .	Tail-like.
Capillaries	. .	Tubes with small bores. A small blood vessel.
Cartilage	. .	Gristle.
Caseine	. .	Cheese. That ingredient in milk which is neither coagulated spontaneously like fibrine, nor by heat like albumen, but by the action of acids alone.
Cataract	. .	Opacity of the lens of the eye, causing blindness if not removed.
Catechu	. .	A dry extract or brown astringent substance.
Cellular	. .	A plant having no spiral vessels, and which is flowerless.
Cerebral	. .	Relating to the brain.
Chlorophyll	.	The green matter of the leaves of vegetables.
Chondrine	. .	The name given to the substance which forms the tissue of cartilage, as it occurs in the ribs, trachea, nose, etc.
Choroid	. .	A term applied to several parts of the body that resemble the chorion.
Chyle	. .	The milk-like fluid into which food is transformed before it is absorbed into the blood.
Cobalt	. .	A mineral of a reddish grey, or greyish white colour, very brittle, of a fine close grain, compact, but easily reducible to powder.
Coccyx	. .	The tail-like termination of the spine.
Copper	. .	A metal of a pale red colour tinged with yellow.
Cornea	. .	The clear glass-like front of the eyeball.
Cretins	. .	A name given to certain deformed and helpless idiots in the Valley of the Alps.
Crucible	. .	A chemical vessel or melting-pot made of earth, and so tempered and baked as to endure heat without melting.

GLOSSARY.

D

Deliquescent	Liquefying in the air.
Derma	The cutis or true skin.
Dextrine	The soluble or gumming matter into which the interior substance of starch globules is convertible by diastase, or by certain acids.
Dry Pile	An electrical instrument.
Dura Mater	A strong membrane lining the interior of the cranium and spinal column.

E

Emphysema	Swelling produced by air, as dropsy is caused by liquid.
Emulsion	A mixture of oil, such as cod liver oil, with water, by aid of gum.
Encephalon	The brain.
Epidemic	A disease attacking a number of people in the same place at one time.
Epidermis	The outermost layer of the skin.
Epiphysis	A process of bone attached by cartilage to the ends of bones, and from which growth takes place.
Equilibrium	Equality of powers.
Erysipelas	Contagious inflammation of the skin, tending to spread.
Excreta	The urine and fæces.

F

Fahr.	The scale of most thermometers used in England.
Fecula	The tasteless matter of plants. Chlorophyll.
Fallopian Tubes	Two trumpet-like canals, about three inches long, passing from the womb to the ovaries.
Fibrin	Albumen of the blood, which solidifies when exposed to the air, and causes coagulation.
Fibrinous	Having or partaking of the nature of fibrin.
Follicle	A minute bag containing some secretion.
Fungi	The name under which botanists class mushrooms, toad-stools, and the microscopic plants called mould, mildew, etc.

G

Ganglial System	An enlargement of a nerve, forming a semi-independent nerve centre.
Gelatinous	Combination of gelatine.
Gluten	A tough, elastic substance, of a greyish colour which becomes brown and brittle by drying.

H

Hæmatemesis	Vomiting blood from the stomach, dark coloured, and often in clots.
Hæmorrhage	A flow of blood.
Hepatic	Relating to the liver.
Hexagonal	Having six sides and six angles.
Hydrogen	An important elementary gas.
Hydro cyanic Acid	Prussic acid.
Hyoid Bone	Shaped like a V, the name of a bone at the root of the tongue.
Hypothesis	A system or theory imagined or assumed to account for what is not understood.

I

Initiation	The act or process of making one acquainted with principles before unknown.

J

Jaundice	Disease of the liver, causing yellowness of the skin.

L

Lacteals	The lymphatic vessels which convey the chyle from the intestinal canal.
Legumin	A peculiar vegetable product obtained from pease.
Ligament	A tough band of fibrous tissue connecting together the bones at the joints.
Lignine	Vegetable fibre. The substance which remains after a plant, or a portion of it, has been treated with water, weak alkaline, and acid solutions with alcohol and ether, in order to dissolve all the matters soluble in these agents.
Luminous	Emitting light.
Lymph	A colourless alkaline fluid found in the lymphatic vessels.

GLOSSARY.

M

Malic Acid	A bibasic acid found in many fruits, particularly in apples.
Mammalia	Relating to the mammals.
Maxiliary Arches	The jaw bones; pertaining to the jaw.
Medullary	Relating to the marrow.
Medusae	A genus of marine radiate animals.
Membrana Tympanum	The ear drum.
Mucus	A viscid fluid of the body, secreted by the mucous membranes.
Mucilage	Gum water.

N

Neurine	The albuminoid matter of a nerve.
Nitrogen	A colourless gas entering largely into the composition of the air we breathe.
Nucleus	The central point of a cell.

O

Oblivion	Forgetfulness; cessation of remembrance.
Ovaries	Two small oval bodies situated on either side of the uterus.
Ossification	Hardening into bone.
Ossific	Having power to ossify, or change membranous substance to bone.
Oxygen	A colourless, odourless gas.

P

Patella	The bone in front of the knee; the knee cap.
Papilla	A small eminence.
Parenchyma	The spongy substance of an organ.
Peristaltic	The worm-like contractions and movements of the intestines in forcing onwards their contents.
Phosphate	A compound of phosphoric acid and a base.
Phosphorus	A non-metallic element used as a nerve tonic and stimulant.
Physiological	The science of the mind, of its various phenomena, affections, and powers.
Pituitary	That secretes phlegm or mucus.

Proteine	. .	A chemical substance obtained from animal or vegetable albumen, fibrin, or caseine, which are all considered to be modifications of it.
Prostate	. .	Heart-shaped gland at the neck of the male bladder.
Pyloric	. .	Pertaining to the pylorus.

R

Retort	. .	A globular vessel with a long neck.

S

Sanguineous	. .	Relating to the blood.
Serous	. .	Pertaining to serum.
Silica	. .	An oxide of silicum.
Stearine	. .	The harder ingredient of animal fats.
Sternum	. .	Breast bone.
Sulphur	. .	A crystalline substance.
Sutures	. .	The joints of bones of the skull.

T

Tarsus	. .	The seven small bones across the instep.
Telephone	. .	An instrument used for far sounding.
Theine	. .	The alkaloid of tea.
Theobromine	.	Oil; the oil extract from cocoa.
Transmutation	.	The change of anything into another substance, or into something of a different nature.

U

Urinary	. .	Pertaining to urine.

V

Vertebræ	. .	The small bones which form the backbone or vertebral column.
Venous	. .	Relating to the veins.
Villi	. .	Small papillæ in the intestine.
Vitreous Humour	.	The glass-like fluid in the eyeball, behind the lens.